Shar[ed] Decision Making in Adult Critical Care

Edited by

Matthew N. Jaffa
Hartford Hospital, Connecticut

David Y. Hwang
Yale University, Connecticut

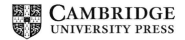
CAMBRIDGE
UNIVERSITY PRESS

CAMBRIDGE
UNIVERSITY PRESS

University Printing House, Cambridge CB2 8BS, United Kingdom

One Liberty Plaza, 20th Floor, New York, NY 10006, USA

477 Williamstown Road, Port Melbourne, VIC 3207, Australia

314–321, 3rd Floor, Plot 3, Splendor Forum, Jasola District Centre,
New Delhi – 110025, India

79 Anson Road, #06–04/06, Singapore 079906

Cambridge University Press is part of the University of Cambridge.

It furthers the University's mission by disseminating knowledge in the pursuit of education, learning, and research at the highest international levels of excellence.

www.cambridge.org
Information on this title: www.cambridge.org/9781108735544
DOI: 10.1017/9781108633246

First published 2021

Printed in the United Kingdom by TJ Books Limited, Padstow Cornwall

A catalogue record for this publication is available from the British Library.

Library of Congress Cataloging-in-Publication Data
Names: Jaffa, Matthew N., editor. | Hwang, David Y., editor.
Title: Shared decision making in adult critical care / edited by Matthew N. Jaffa, David Y. Hwang.
Description: Cambridge, United Kingdom ; New York, NY : Cambridge University
    Press, 2021. | Includes bibliographical references and index.
Identifiers: LCCN 2020051656 (print) | LCCN 2020051657 (ebook) |
    ISBN 9781108735544 (paperback) | ISBN 9781108633246 (epub)
Subjects: MESH: Critical Care–methods | Clinical Decision-Making | Decision Making, Shared
    | Patient Participation | Professional-Patient Relations | Professional-Family Relations
Classification: LCC RC86.7 (print) | LCC RC86.7 (ebook) | NLM WX 218 |
    DDC 616.02/8–dc23
LC record available at https://lccn.loc.gov/2020051656
LC ebook record available at https://lccn.loc.gov/2020051657

ISBN 978-1-108-73554-4 Paperback

Contents

Contributors

Catherine L. Auriemma, MD
Fellow, Division of Pulmonary and Critical Care Medicine, Hospital of the University of Pennsylvania; Post-Doctoral Fellow, Palliative and Advanced Illness Center; Associate Fellow, Leonard Davis Center for Health Economics

Christopher Bryant, MD
Resident, Department of Neurology, UT Southwestern

Elizabeth Carroll, MD
Resident, Department of Neurology, NYU Langone Medical Center

Philip Choi, MD
Assistant Professor of Internal Medicine, Division of Pulmonary Critical Care Medicine, University of Michigan

Katharine R. Colton, MD
Fellow, Neurocritical Care, Department of Neurology, Northwestern University, Feinberg School of Medicine

Claire J. Creutzfeldt, MD
Associate Professor, Department of Neurology, University of Washington, Harborview Hospital

Timothy M. Dempsey, MD, MPH
Division of Pulmonary and Critical Care Medicine, Mayo Clinic

Connie Ge, BA
Department of Neurology, University of Massachusetts School of Medicine

Adeline L. Goss, MD
Neurohospitalist Fellow, Department of Neurology, University of California, San Francisco

Mitra Haeri, MD, MBE
Resident, Department of Neurology, University of Maryland School of Medicine

David Y. Hwang, MD, FAAN, FCCM, FNCS
Associate Professor, Division of Neurocritical Care and Emergency Neurology, Department of Neurology, Yale School of Medicine

Matthew N. Jaffa, DO
Neurointensivist, Associate Director NeuroRecovery Clinic, Section of Neurocritical Care, Department of Neurology, Ayer Neuroscience Institute, Hartford Hospital; Assistant Professor of Neurology, University of Connecticut School of Medicine

Joshua B. Kayser, MD, MPH, MBE, FCCM
Associate Professor of Clinical Medicine and Medical Ethics, Division of Pulmonary, Allergy and Critical Care, Department of Medicine; Department of Medical Ethics and Health Policy, Perelman School of Medicine, University of Pennsylvania; Section Chief, Medical Critical Care; Director, Medical Intensive Care Unit; Co-Director, Pulmonary Hypertension Program, Cpl. Michael J. Crescenz VA Medical Center

Angelos Kolias, MD, PhD, FRCS (SN)
Clinical Lecturer, Division of Neurosurgery, Department of Clinical Neurosciences, Addenbrooke's Hospital and University of Cambridge

Jacqueline M. Kruser, MD, MS
Assistant Professor, Department of Medicine, Division of Allergy, Pulmonary, and Critical Care, University of Wisconsin School of Medicine and Public Health

Barnaby Lewin, MA, MRCP, FRCA, FFICM, DTMH
Senior Resident Physician CTICU, National University Hospital

Ariane Lewis, MD
Director of Neurocritical Care; Associate Professor of Neurology and Neurosurgery, NYU Langone Medical Center

Carolina B. Maciel, MD, MSCR
Assistant Professor of Neurology and Neurosurgery; Director of Research, Division of Neurocritical Care, University of Florida

Chris Marcellino, MD
Neurocritical Care Fellow, Neurologic Surgery Chief Resident, Mayo Clinic

Evie G. Marcolini, MD, FAAEM, FACEP, FCCM
Associate Professor of Emergency Medicine and Neurology, Geisel School of Medicine at Dartmouth; Board of Directors, American Academy of Emergency Medicine

Paul McCarthy, MD
Director, Cardiovascular Critical Care, Critical Care Medicine and Nephrology; Assistant Professor of Medicine, WVU Heart & Vascular Institute

Jessica McFarlin, MD
Associate Professor of Neurology, Division Chief Palliative and Supportive Care, University of Kentucky College of Medicine

Melissa Motta, MD
Assistant Professor, Division of Neurocritical Care and Emergency Neurology, Department of Neurology, Program in Trauma, University of Maryland School of Medicine

Susanne Muehlschlegel, MD, MPH
Associate Professor, Departments of Neurology, Anesthesia/Critical Care and Surgery, University of Massachusetts School of Medicine

Alejandro A. Rabinstein, MD
Professor of Neurology; Director, Neuroscience ICU, Mayo Clinic

Kollengode Ramanathan, MBBS, FCICM, FCCP
Senior Consultant, Department of Cardiac, Thoracic and Vascular Surgery, National University Heart Centre; Director, ICU Fellowship Programme, National University Hospital; Assistant Professor, Department of Surgery, Yong Loo Lin School of Medicine, National University of Singapore

Joshua Rolnick, MD, JD, MS
Staff Physician, Philadelphia VA Medical Center; Clinical Assistant Professor of Medicine, University of Pennsylvania School of Medicine

Michael A. Rubin, MD, MA, FAAN
Associate Professor, Neurology and Neurosurgery, Division of Neurocritical Care; Chair, UT Southwestern Clinical Ethics; Neurology Quality and Safety Lead, Peter J. O'Donnell, Jr. Brain Institute, UT Southwestern Medical Center

Nneka O. Sederstrom, PhD, MPH, MA, FCCP, FCCM
Director, Clinical Ethics Department, Children's Hospitals and Clinics of Minnesota

Hassan Suleiman, MD
Fellow, Department of Nephrology, West Virginia University

Stephen Trevick, MD
Neurohospitalist and Neurointensivist, Northwest Neurology; Psychiatrist, Northwestern Memorial Hospital

Alison E. Turnbull, DVM, MPH, PhD
Associate Professor, Division of Pulmonary and Critical Care Medicine, Department of Medicine, School of Medicine; Department of Epidemiology, Bloomberg School of Public Health, Johns Hopkins University

Alexandra Wichmann, MD
Resident, Department of Internal Medicine, Texas Tech University Health Sciences Center

Matthew Wilson, MD
Fellow, Division of Pulmonary Critical Care Medicine, University of Michigan

Michael E. Wilson, MD
Division of Pulmonary and Critical Care Medicine, Robert D. and Patricia E. Kern Center for the Science of Health Care Delivery, Knowledge and Evaluation Research Unit, Mayo Clinic

Sonya E. Zhou, BS
Department of Neurology, Yale School of Medicine

Preface

Decisions about life, quality of life, and death are routine in critical care practice. To promote the ethical principle of patient autonomy, clinicians often find themselves incorporating their medical expertise into value-laden conversations with patients and families of incapacitated patients – with regard to whether clinical care plans are consistent with patients' wishes, or the best approximation thereof.

Guiding patients and families through these shared decisions can be difficult, not necessarily because of detailed technical knowledge needed to understand how interventions work in the intensive care unit (ICU), but because of the uncertainty of what ICU interventions might achieve at any given time for a certain patient and the challenges of conveying difficult news to overwhelmed patients and families – whether that news is certain or uncertain. ICU teams are generally large and multidisciplinary, and although the complexity of such conversations warrants a clinician with expertise and compassion guiding them, it is not infrequent that these conversations are led by clinical trainees who build close relationships with patients and families, but who may not have a wealth of experience from which to draw.

In this context, our hope is that all critical care clinicians – but especially students, trainees, and those early in their independent careers – will find this easy-to-read book on shared decision-making in ICUs to be both useful and practical. The first four introductory chapters of this book cover some basic principles that apply to a wide variety of scenarios – assessing what types of decision are appropriate opportunities for shared decision-making, how involved a patient's family wishes to be in decisions, how best to present quantitative information, and how to optimize family discussions. The middle 11 chapters cover specific, common clinical scenarios in critical care that require clinicians to weave together their basic medical knowledge with shared decision-making approaches. These chapters are all case based and provide recommended frameworks for approach. The reader will find that some core principles are repeated throughout these chapters, but also that the chapter authors highlight key references and statistics that may help clinicians in planning their discussions with patients and families. A fair number of these chapters are neurologic in nature; this fact admittedly in part represents our editorial bias as neurointensivists, but also is an acknowledgment that the degree of neurologic recovery is often a key factor in goals-of-care decisions made in critical care.

This book ends with a few chapters on a potpourri of related topics – advance directives, care of the unbefriended patient, and incorporating palliative care consultants into the ICU. We have also included a chapter on how researchers grapple with the difficult question of how best to measure "success" for ICU shared decisions. One could potentially argue that the final chapter on discussions regarding brain death is perhaps a bit outside what one considers a truly "shared" decision – because death by neurologic criteria is still legal death. Yet, communicating such a concept to families is challenging in its own right, and many principles that apply to shared decision-making conversations apply in brain death conversations as well.

We note that the chapters in this book were nearly all written before the onset of the worldwide novel coronavirus disease-2019 (COVID-19) pandemic. The concerns during the height of the pandemic – that ICU resources even in resource-rich environments would possibly need to be widely rationed, that hospitals needed revised protocols for determining code statuses for patients with COVID-19, and that prolonged strict visitor restriction policies were necessary – became multiple barriers to our field's standard methods of promoting shared decision-making. Some of the principles of this book are preserved whether one is having discussions with families in person or via phone/video conference; others require significant flexibility. We acknowledge as well that still others may be profoundly affected by the risk COVID-19 presents to clinicians themselves (i.e., how a clinician discusses offering cardiopulmonary resuscitation for COVID-19–positive patients with a poor chance of survival).

Our hope is that, by the time this book is published, the risk of virus transmission will be lower than it was in the spring and summer of 2020 and the families that we all depend on so much will be at ICU patients' bedsides with increased frequency. But even if that is unfortunately not the case, we hope that this book is a reminder – especially to those entering the practice of medicine amid a pandemic – that shared decision-making is not merely an optional approach to be practiced by clinicians when convenient, but that the principle of incorporating patient's values into decisions that ideally require knowledge of them is an immutable tenet of ethical and high-quality critical care practice.

Chapter 1

When Does Shared Decision-Making Apply in Adult Critical Care?

Matthew N. Jaffa and David Y. Hwang

Shared decision-making in medicine has been defined by multiple professional societies as "a collaborative process that allows patients, or their surrogates, and clinicians to make health-care decisions together, taking into account the best scientific evidence available, as well as the patient's values, goals and preferences."[1] This definition incorporates several important ethical principles simultaneously; it acknowledges the importance of patient autonomy. Patient autonomy incorporates a patient's personal values and respects the degree to which he or she might wish to be involved in a decision about his or her own medical care.[2] It also recognizes the critical role of clinicians as experts in actively advising patients about the benefits and risks of their available treatment options and in designing treatment plans to align with patients' ultimate goals and preferences.

1.1 Challenges with Practicing Shared Decision-Making in Critical Care

At its core, the practice of shared decision-making centers on informed collaboration and mutual deliberation between clinicians and patients.[3] In emergency department and critical care environments, there are multiple barriers that prevent collaboration and mutual deliberation with patients from occurring easily. Patients and families are often meeting clinicians for the first time, with relatively little time to build trust. Important decisions often must be made in a time-sensitive manner. Many patients, especially in intensive care units (ICUs), lack capacity to participate in or make decisions. Those patients who do have capacity may nevertheless have significant communication barriers, such as being mechanically ventilated. Clear and specific scientific evidence regarding benefits and risks may not exist for many important decisions that need to be made. However, despite these recognized barriers, clinicians in emergency rooms and ICUs must strive to practice shared decision-making to the best degree possible when situations call for it, because of its strong ethical justification.

For a patient to demonstrate the "capacity" to make choices related to the direction of their medical care, he or she must have the ability to (1) integrate information about their illness and treatment, (2) consider the nature of various alternatives and their consequences, (3) rationally question all information that is presented, and (4) communicate a decision that is consistent with their own personal values.[4] Intubated patients may use communication boards if they remain awake on minimal amounts of sedation, although aphasic patients may require additional assessment and teamwork with speech pathologists to delineate a means for clear communication.[5] Advances in technology may even allow for patients with neuromuscular weakness or locked-in syndrome to communicate via eye-gaze systems and newer devices such as brain–computer interfaces. However, in the ICU, the patient's being unable to participate in collaboration and mutual deliberation is more often the rule rather than the exception.

When an ICU patient is unable to participate in shared decision-making, advance care planning documentation may already exist that can provide insight to a patient's preferences.[6,7] However, most adults in the United States do not have a completed advanced directive. For those who have completed one, the details have often not been shared with their families or the persons they have appointed to be responsible.[8] Even the most clearly delineated advanced directives are generally unable to cover every possible situation that may occur and often only address concerns related to extreme medical futility.

These limitations in pre-existing care planning for incapacitated patients more often than not require that surrogate decision makers enter into the clinician–patient relationship as partners to help decide on important aspects and directions of emergency and ICU care. However, even if a proper surrogate (or surrogates) is identified, the process of surrogate decision-making can be fraught with challenges.[9] A surrogate may happen to not be an adequate judge of what a patient's wishes would have been in any specific situation, whether the surrogate realizes it or not. Several studies have revealed surrogates to be imperfect predictors of patient preferences, overestimating their desire for life-prolonging interventions.[10,11] Surrogates may also incorporate their own preferences and personal factors in decision-making, aside from simply exercising substituted judgment on behalf of the incapacitated patient.[12]

The fact that ICU clinicians work with surrogate decision makers on a daily basis does not necessarily mitigate the practical challenges with shared decision-making outlined in this chapter. Because this book discusses general strategies for approaching many of these practical challenges and outlines considerations in certain common specific scenarios, it is prudent to briefly review examples of ICU situations in which shared decision-making may apply and those in which it may not.

1.2 Situations in Which Principles of Shared Decision-Making Apply in ICUs

Hundreds of decisions are made daily in the ICU, many of which patients and families may only be aware of if participating in bedside rounds or if constantly at the bedside. Which ICU decisions warrant collaboration and deliberation?

The shared decision-making approach is most relevant regarding those care decisions that are truly affected by a patient's individual preferences, goals, and attitudes toward acceptable quality of life. Conditions where uncertainty exists regarding both survival and functional recovery routinely warrant collaboration and deliberation among clinicians and patients/surrogates to explore treatment options that are based on scientific evidence in the context of the patient's perceived preferences.[13] However, every admission to an ICU can be considered an opportunity for clinicians to initiate discussions with patients and their families regarding patients' goals of care, as well as preferences and values, especially before medical emergencies occur, where a patient might later be rendered incapacitated. Importantly, routine decisions in patient care that are not typically value laden – such as which laboratory tests to order, which antibiotics to use to treat a urinary tract infection, etc. – can and should be made in general by treating clinicians based on consensus best practices and evidence-based implementation.

Table 1.1 provides examples of health-care decisions encountered in the critical care unit that are ideal for the practice of shared decision-making.

Table 1.1 Examples of decisions appropriate for shared decision-making[1]

1. Whether to undergo decompressive hemicraniectomy in a patient with malignant stroke and cerebral swelling.
2. Whether to pursue ongoing weaning efforts at ventilator facility or transition to palliative care for a patient with advanced chronic obstructive pulmonary disease having failed several attempts at ventilator weaning in the ICU.
3. Whether a patient's quality of life is sufficiently satisfying that she or he would want life-sustaining treatment when a life-threatening event occurs.
4. Whether to initiate renal replacement therapy in a patient with significant volume overload who has terminal cancer.
5. Whether to implement extracorporeal membrane oxygenation in a 90-year-old patients with loss of consciousness owing to pulmonary embolus while on the golf course.

Reprinted from Kon A, et al. Shared decision making in ICUs: An American College of Critical Care Medicine and American Thoracic Society Policy Statement, *Crit Care Med.* vol. 44(1), 2016, with permission from Wolters Kluwer Health.

Several chapters of this book address potential challenges with the overall processes of shared decision-making in ICUs, and others discuss specific common clinical scenarios, such as the ones presented in Section 1.2 and Table 1.1 and suggest approaches for using available outcome data to guide individualized discussions with patients and surrogates. Implementing shared decision-making in critical care scenarios can be complex and time consuming, and – despite clinicians' best efforts – situations can at times result in intractable conflict with patients and families that may be challenging and frustrating to resolve. In the face of these and other challenges, we hope that this book will help to provide a framework to aid readers in their own best efforts to collaborate and deliberate with patients and families when moments arise that call for shared decisions.

References

1. A.A. Kon, J.E. Davidson, W. Morrison, M. Danis, D.B. White, American College of Critical Care Medicine, et al. Shared decision making in ICUs: an American College of Critical Care Medicine and American Thoracic Society Policy Statement. *Critical Care Medicine* 2016; 44(1): 188–201.

2. P.A. Ubel, K.A. Scherr, A. Fagerlin. Autonomy: what's shared decision making have to do with it? *American Journal of Bioethics*, 2018; 18(2): W11–W12.

3. A. Edwards, G. Elwyn. *Shared Decision Making in Health Care: Achieving Evidence-Based Patient Choice*, 3rd ed. Oxford: Oxford University Press; 2016.

4. P.S. Appelbaum, T. Grisso. Assessing patients' capacities to consent to treatment. *New England Journal of Medicine* 1988; 319(25): 1635–8.

5. L. Patak, A. Gawlinski, N.I. Fung, L. Doering, J. Berg, E.A. Henneman. Communication boards in critical care: patients' views. *Applied Nursing Research: ANR* 2006; 19(4): 182–90.

6. V.P. Tilden, S.W. Tolle, C.A. Nelson, J. Fields. Family decision-making to withdraw life-sustaining treatments from hospitalized patients. *Nursing Research* 2001; 50(2): 105–15.

7. A. Majesko, S.Y. Hong, L. Weissfeld, D.B. White. Identifying family members who may struggle in the role of surrogate decision maker. *Critical Care Medicine* 2012; 40(8): 2281–6.

8. W. Benson, N. Aldrich. *Advance Care Planning: Ensuring Your Wishes Are Known and Honored If You Are Unable to Speak for Yourself, Critical Issue Brief.* Atlanta: Centers for Disease Control and Prevention; 2012.

9. D. Wendler, A. Rid. Systematic review: the effect on surrogates of making treatment decisions for others. *Annals of Internal Medicine* 2011; 154(5): 336–46.

10. A.B. Seckler, D.E. Meier, M. Mulvihill, B.E. Cammer Paris. Substituted judgment: how accurate are proxy predictions? *Annals of Internal Medicine* 1991; 115(2): 92–8.

11. J. Suhl, P. Simons, T. Reedy, T. Garrick. Myth of substituted judgment: surrogate decision making regarding life support is unreliable. *Archives of Internal Medicine* 1994; 154(1): 90–6.

12. D. Brudney. Choosing for another: beyond autonomy and best interests. *Hastings Center Report* 2009; 39(2): 31–7.

13. C. Charles, T. Whelan, A. Gafni. What do we mean by partnership in making decisions about treatment? *BMJ* 1999; 319(7212): 780–2.

Chapter 2

How Much Does the Family Want to Be Involved in Decision-Making?

Christopher Bryant and Michael A. Rubin

As advancements in medical therapy improve survival, we are confronted with more patients who either cannot communicate or lack decisional capacity, leaving a more common dependency on collaborations with surrogate decision makers. Accompanying these advancements also come radically more complex scenarios to consider that require us to occasionally compromise between quality of life and longevity of life. For instance, modalities such as continuous renal replacement therapy, extracorporeal membrane oxygenation, left ventricular assist devices, and organ transplantation can certainly extend the lives of their recipients, but at a cost of potential complications, time in the hospital, and variable success. Further, the scale between physician-directed decision-making and medical consumerism is weighing heavier toward giving patients a wider breadth of decisional authority in their health care, and the intensive care unit (ICU) is no exception. The recognition of the importance of autonomous decision-making in the latter half of the twentieth century created a need to establish the shared medical decision-making model that incorporates the values and choices of patients with the medical expertise of the physician, as discussed elsewhere in this text (see Chapter 1, When Does Shared Decision-Making Apply in Adult Critical Care?). A natural extension to the increasingly used shared decision-making model requires that we make reasonable efforts to seek the collaboration with surrogate decision-makers when the patient is unable to represent themselves.[1]

Shared decision-making and the expansion of consumerism may be a novel idea for families. Although the ethics literature often focuses on the importance of adjusting to the contemporary paradigm of shared medical decision-making, we must also consider the other half of the equation. We unknowingly make a significant leap forward when we assume that all patients and surrogates will embrace this methodology or even agree to participate in this model. Some patients might even prefer a more traditional method of decision-making, wherein the physician is the sole decision maker, and find it uncomfortable or odd to be given choices that they think are the domain of the physician. In fact, only about one-half of surrogates prefer to play a role in medical decision-making.[2] We must come to the realization that, if we are going to elevate the importance of autonomy, we ought to include the decision maker's right to forgo elements of that autonomy if it meets their needs. In contrast, other patients may not wish to yield much decision-making at all and believe they should be given every potential option, even those that the physician's experience and the evidence would suggest are very likely to cause more harm than benefit.

There are some psychological subtleties to the literature on this subject; for instance, gender, religiosity, and trust in medicine are associated with certain expectations from surrogates regarding their role.[2] These details do not capture the full spectrum of surrogate qualities and preference; every patient and surrogate should be approached initially with an open mind with regard to their desired input in the decision-making for the patient. As the provider–surrogate relationship develops, over time this approach can be fine-tuned to better fit individual circumstances. For example, an engineer might prefer more detail-oriented data and clearly enumerated options, whereas a spiritually oriented person may only want to be involved in purely value-laden questions. The only way to differentiate these two would be to invest enough time in understanding their background.

Although presuming the extent to which surrogates want decision-making roles before fostering a partnership is ill-advised, the content of the decision definitely changes both surrogate and provider opinion on where the responsibility lies. Distinguishing minor decisions from major decisions is important to help clarify for which issues most surrogates would like to have input. On average, there are about nine decisions per patient per daily rounds.[3] It would be inefficient and overwhelming to surrogates if all of these decisions were addressed with them, and the majority of the decisions would likely best be determined from medical expertise alone.

Within the many decisions to be made is an intermingling of technical decisions and those with value-laden implications. For instance, consider intubation. The decision to place a breathing tube is a heavily value-laden one; therefore, patient goals of care – if they can be obtained – should be equally important to the medical indication to intubate. For a patient with respiratory failure, intubation and ventilation are a commitment to a care path that is very different than if they are forgone. A divide between a likely death and potentially living with a disability or a protracted hospital course is created. By contrast, the decision as to which size endotracheal tube to place lacks a component of personal value and depends on patient mechanics and provider expertise. Distinguishing value-laden decisions from technical decisions can aid providers in addressing the appropriate topics in family discussions and focus on what really matters with regards to surrogate decision-making. This practice can also help to keep surrogates from being overwhelmed with choices and allow them more time to speak on value-laden decisions. Typically, surrogates are not concerned with what size endotracheal tube the team would like to use for an intubation, no more than a plane passenger wants to be consulted on what elevation their commercial airline should choose to cruise.

Occasionally, a surrogate may request a provider fill a more paternalistic role with a question such as, "What would you do?" This question is a direct invitation to contribute more to the value-laden component of decision-making. If done at the behest of the surrogate, there is no harm in suggesting what we as physicians believe is best; it can be a good exercise in empathy as well. We should be careful to acknowledge that we are applying our personal values to the situation, however. Similar to a provider caring for their own loved one, mixing medical practice with personal relationships can compromise the quality of care. Alternatively, these situations can be good opportunities to help surrogates bridge the gap between medical care and their loved one's values. Identifying specific qualities about the patient, in conjunction with an educated discussion on prognosis, can clarify how certain interventions will affect each individual patient. It is not uncommon for surrogates to misunderstand the downstream reality of medical interventions, so coupling that knowledge with pertinent examples may help to decrease the confusion.[4]

Of course, some surrogates are sincerely looking for a direct answer to the question, especially if they have a more traditional view of the role of physicians and expect a paternalistic approach. They could also be trying to subconsciously avoid the psychological trauma of making these decisions, or they just feel lost in the fray. Ensuring that surrogates are at least approached with the responsibility of shared decision-making is an opportunity that should not be missed, because there are advantages to surrogate involvement in patient care that extend beyond medical decision-making.

From a practical standpoint, family and surrogates can be a valuable resource in a noncommunicative patient's presentation when gathering the history. Establishing the details of patient care and values early on with surrogates can help to guide decisions if the surrogate is unavailable to discuss medical interventions in a critical moment. The duration of stay for patients in an ICU as well as mortality rates may be decreased by increasing time spent communicating with family about decisions.[5] Common ICU-related complications, such as ICU delirium, can be mitigated with increased family presence by helping to reorient the patient, ensure they have sensory aids if needed, and provide them with a sense of familiarity.[6] Family members frequently assist nurses with routine care of the patient; simply being there to help turn or clean their loved ones can alleviate burden on health-care workers.[7] Of course, after the patient leaves the ICU, the family may play a primary role as health-care provider at home, and involving them early on in routine care can help to prepare them for a softer transition out of the hospital and strengthen their discharge training.

Having a loved one ill in an ICU can easily consume the lives of surrogates. Although their presence can be invaluable to providers, it does not come without its own sharp edge. Surrogates who help in decision-making are susceptible to symptoms of post-traumatic stress and ultimately are at risk to develop post-traumatic stress disorder.[8] Higher rates were associated with family members who felt the information they received was incomplete, if their relative died in the ICU, if they died after end-of-life decisions, if they shared in the decision-making, and most of all if the members shared in end-of-life decisions.[8] The latter part of these data act as an apparent counterweight to much of the discussion presented. Providers need to understand the psychological toll that these conversations can have on family; a routine discussion for them may be the moment that wakes a spouse in the middle of the night for years to come. To what extent are providers responsible for the well-being of surrogates? Of course, patient care is the primary concern for physicians, but it is unfortunate that this goal can be at odds with surrogate well-being and that there is not a better compromise to address this situation.

To a certain extent, it should be expected that families who watch their loved ones endure time and possibly death in an ICU undergo some psychological stress; however, more work needs to be done to address surrogate stress, because their input is increasingly incorporated into patient care. For instance, earlier involvement in medical decision-making before end-of-life decisions are associated with an easier time coping when the decision has to be made.[9] Careful language can help to reframe the conversation – instead of presenting the decision to "let the patient die," it can be said to "alleviate suffering," or "allow the natural disease process to run its course," or another softer alternative.[9] When surrogates know a patient's preference ahead of time, they will likely have a less difficult time with tough decisions, highlighting the importance for primary care providers to encourage patients with chronic illnesses to discuss their preferences early with potential surrogate decision makers.[9] Continuity of care and having one provider be the primary resource for surrogates to turn to is also associated with improved surrogate well-being.[9] And, to further emphasize the importance of establishing a relationship with surrogates and coming to know their preferred level of input, some surrogates feel empowered when contributing to medical decision-making as a form of coping. In fact, it could be particularly distressing for a surrogate who expects to have their hand on the tiller to watch their loved one's health roll aimlessly in the waves while they stand powerless on the shore. It is important to identify those who may benefit from feeling more in control and accommodating them as appropriate. These measures can help to attenuate extraneous stress on family members and surrogates in our increasingly collaborative health-care environment.

The ever-changing landscape of medicine carves different challenges for current and future providers. A combination of changing attitudes on how medical decisions should be made and shifting patient scenarios has culminated in a reliance on individuals other than the patient to participate in the health care of their families. Juggling the health and relationship of a single patient can be a daunting task, let alone a series of family members, all with their own unique ideas of how medicine works and what they believe their and the provider's role should be. For the reasons summarized, family and surrogate involvement will be an increasingly used collaboration and, if done well, can provide useful advantages to providers and patients alike. The individuals who speak on behalf of our patients should not be seen as another obstacle to finishing the day's work, but as one more opportunity to provide good health care to patients. They should also be seen as ends in themselves, and more should be done to address their traumas when they choose to be on the front lines with providers as their loved ones are critically ill or dying. Providers will need to remain agile in meeting the spectrum of expectations from family members; there is no single approach that provides universal success. Ultimately, surrogates should be encouraged to involve themselves in decision-making as much as they feel comfortable and as much as is medically safe and reasonable, with the shared goal of the patient's best interest.

References

1. A.A. Kon, J.E. Davidson, W. Morrison, D.B. White. Shared decision making in intensive care units: executive summary of the American College of Critical Care Medicine and American Thoracic Society Policy Statement. *American Journal of Respiratory Critical Care Medicine* 2016; 44(1): 188–201.

2. S.K. Johnson, C.A. Bautista, S.Y. Hong, L. Weissfeld, D.B. White. An empirical study of surrogates' preferred level of control over value-laden life support decisions in intensive care units. *American Journal of Respiratory Critical Care Medicine* 2011; 183(7): 915–21.

3. M.S. McKenzie, C.L. Auriemma, J. Olenik, E. Cooney, N.B. Gabler, S.D. Halpern. An observational study of decision making by medical intensivists. *Critical Care Medicine* 2015; 43(8): 1660–8.

4. E. Azoulay, S. Chevret, G. Leleu, F. Pochard, M. Barboteu, C. Adrie, et al. Half the families of intensive care unit patients experience inadequate communication with physicians. *Critical Care Medicine* 2000; 28(8): 3044–9.

5. C.M. Lilly, L.A. Sonna, K.J. Haley, A.F. Massaro. Intensive communication: four-year follow-up from a clinical practice study. *Critical Care Medicine* 2003; 31(5): S394–9.

6. R.G. Rosa, T.F. Tonietto, D.B. da Silva, F.A. Gutierres, A.M. Ascoli. Effectiveness and safety of an extended ICU visitation model for delirium prevention: a before and after study. *Critical Care Medicine* 2017; 45(10): 1660–7.

7. J.L. McAdam, S. Arai, K.A. Puntillo. Unrecognized contributions of families in the intensive care unit. *Intensive Care Med* 2008; 34(6): 1097–101.

8. E. Azoulay, F. Pochard, N. Kentish-Barnes, S. Chevret, J. Aboab. Risk of post-traumatic stress symptoms in family members of intensive care unit patients. *American Journal of Respiratory Critical Care Medicine* 2005; 171(9): 987–94.

9. E. Vig, H. Starks, J. Taylor, E. Hopley, K. Fryer-Edwards. Surviving surrogate decision-making: what helps and hampers the experience of making medical decisions for others. *Journal of General Internal Medicine* 2007; 22(9): 1274–9.

Show Me the Data

Tips for Discussing Numerical Risk in Critical Care

Mitra Haeri and Melissa Motta

Shared decision-making involves using the best scientific evidence available to make a choice together with the patient or their surrogate, while weighing the options against the patient's values, preferences, and goals. A lion's share of the process, therefore, must be devoted to conveying the clinical information and the science surrounding the available options to the patient, or their surrogate, as is often the case in critical care. There are multiple pitfalls to be aware of when conveying numerical risk to patients and families that can impede their decision-making ability. First, numeracy – an aspect of literacy that deals specifically with understanding numbers – can be very poor, even among highly educated people, creating a barrier to comprehending clinical information. Second, the manner in which numerical data are presented can easily manipulate the cognitive biases of patients and their surrogates, limiting their autonomy. Third, clinicians may often present their *interpretation* of numerical risk rather than the actual data, corrupting the step in shared decision-making where we elicit values and preferences from the patient, imprinting their own values instead. In this Chapter, we explore these issues and discuss ways to optimize the presentation of numerical information.

3.1 Understanding the Difficulty of Numeracy

At the heart of many critical care conversations is information sharing and prognostication – patients and families want to know what to expect as a serious illness takes its course. Numerical risk ends up being a large part of these discussions (i.e., "What are the exact chances my loved one is ever going to walk again?"). However, if patients and families do not understand the information being presented, it would be suboptimal to have it used as the basis of their supposedly "informed" decisions.

Leiter et al.[1] uncovered in their study of numeracy in the intensive care setting that almost one-half of participants had low numeracy and had difficulty with basic questions with numbers (e.g. "Which confers the greatest risk, 1%, 5%, or 10%?"). Many of these participants were highly educated, with 70%

of those considered low numeracy surrogates having completed at least some college. Numerous cases given were exactly the type of statements that clinicians present to surrogates and patients every day; for example, "A 50-year-old woman presents with an intracerebral hemorrhage score of 2, which predicts a 74% chance of survival. What do you think the chances are that this patient will survive?" with participants being asked to complete a fill-in-the-blank of the percent likelihood, from 0% to 99%. Almost 50% of participants answered incorrectly. Numerical risk is, therefore, extremely difficult to communicate effectively, recognizing that a large portion of people do not fully understand its true implications.

Adding to this challenge, people do not necessarily have insight regarding their own numeracy skills, although these skills factor heavily into how we make decisions. Even though many people have low numeracy, they nevertheless often prefer to receive numerical rather than qualitative information, often placing more trust in physicians who present numbers rather than verbal descriptions. Higher levels of trust do correlate with decision-makers with higher levels of numeracy.[2]

Although patients with greater numeracy are in general more likely to actually use numbers in making their decisions, those with lesser numeracy are also more likely to use other factors, such as emotions and trust in the healthcare system.[3] Patients and surrogates may have a lack of insight into this tendency, a fact that may also contribute to communication issues in the clinical setting.

Finally, providers themselves can have a difficult time with interpreting and using numbers in their clinical practice and their conversations with patients and families.[4] There is a great deal of uncertainty in medicine, and extrapolating choices for a single patient based on statistics – even assuming the best quality evidence, i.e., multicenter double-blind randomized control trial, is a challenging task. When the evidence provides clear guidelines, clinicians still have to use their own judgment to make treatment decisions, understanding that statistics cannot necessarily be applied to individual events or patients.

3.2 Cognitive Biases

Aside from issues of actually understanding the numbers, human cognition is governed in large part by unconscious, rapid, gut reaction judgments, including our cognitive biases (Table 3.1).[5] Clinicians can exploit these cognitive biases to guide patients' and families' decisions toward outcomes they have deemed to be in the best interest of their patient(s).

Framing is a common way in which biases are used; i.e., the same information is described differently and influences people to make one choice or another. Patients and families may choose different treatment options if the

Table 3.1. Examples of cognitive biases

Default effects	People are more likely to stay with preset options than they are to actively change those options; e.g., the default settings on your computer or smartphone.
Framing effects	People respond differently to equivalent information depending on how it is presented; e.g., people will purchase more fuel if the gas prices are discounted for those paying with cash rather than up-charged for those paying with credit.
Optimism bias	People tend to believe they are better off than they actually are; e.g., smokers tend to believe that they are less likely to develop cancer than nonsmokers do.
Priming	People are more likely to recall certain things or act certain ways when subtly prompted to do so; e.g., people who read a list of words related to old age are likely to perform a subsequent task more slowly than they would have otherwise.

prognosis is described as having a 90% survival rate rather than as having a 10% mortality rate, even though these statements are equivalent. Peters et al.[3] found that people with lower numeracy skills were actually more susceptible to framing effects. Indeed, stating a risk as a percentage versus a frequency can have implications on the perceived risk. Moreover, using qualitative statements such as a "high probability of death" can lead to a wider range of interpretations.[6]

Cognitive biases are an important driver of human behavior, and it is vitally important for clinicians to be aware of them when discussing these important life-and-death matters with their patients and families.

When presenting numbers and data to patients and families, one must keep in mind that what they may consider a "good" outcome may be very different than what the clinician, or even the medical community, views as an acceptable outcome. The modified Rankin Scale (mRS), for example, is a widely used functional outcome measure that describes the level of neurologic disability that patients experience (see Chapter 11, Decompressive Craniectomy for Stroke Patients). However, often when talking about "good" outcomes, the scores 0–3, ranging from no disability to moderate disability (i.e., requiring some help but able to walk without assistance) are used; and when talking about "poor" outcomes, scores of 4–6, ranging from moderately severe disability (i.e., unable to walk without assistance and unable to attend to bodily needs without assistance, to death) are used. Although death, an mRS of 6, is obviously a poor outcome, it is much less obvious that an mRS of 4 might also be, given that many patients who recover from devastating illnesses go on to require a cane or walker, and may need help with some of their activities of daily living. Many people may consider themselves very fortunate to survive a devastating stroke or traumatic brain injury with an mRS of 4, and to present convincing data that frames this outcome as poor may not be fair to decision makers. As such, it is important to note that much of the evidence-based data available is defined using similar scales with relatively arbitrary values delineating "good" from "bad."

Even in cases where *a priori* statements indicate that patients would not want to live with any type of disability, many post-illness disabled survivors consider themselves to have an excellent quality of life – a situation known as the "disability paradox." Although there are many reasons one might question this paradox's validity – including simply that the *most* severely disabled patients are unlikely to be able to report their quality of life, which may in fact be very poor – there are an equal number of real-world examples demonstrating its truth when we look.[7,8]

3.3 Methods to Improve Insight If Numbers Are Presented

If one decides to present numbers during shared decision-making discussions, there are several approaches one can take to optimize the presentation of quantitative information to patients and families.[3] Peters et al.[3] first suggest distilling what is presented to only the most relevant information. Too much information can be confounding and contribute negatively to an already confusing situation. They also recommend reducing the number of calculations required. For example, using a common denominator like 5/100 and 1/100 instead of 1/20 and 1/200 can help to increase comprehension. Along these same lines, advanced statistical concepts such as confidence intervals or number needed to treat may be helpful and even critical for accuracy in many situations, but these concepts need to be presented with care.[9]

Research suggests that visual displays (Figure 3.1) can be helpful (e.g., risks associated with tissue plasminogen activator). These visual displays should represent the total population of interest as well as persons affected.[9]

Framing effects can be mitigated by preparing clinicians with questions one might ask to help patients and surrogates make decisions that align with their values.[9] For example, to de-bias the effect of default options, one should ask people to think of reasons for their decision or even to have them write their reasons out. Doing so requires people to weigh the alternatives more evenly with the default option. Similarly, for the framing effect, studies have demonstrated that asking people to elaborate on their decisions decreases the effect.[10]

Other de-biasing studies addressing the framing effect showed that people who were primed to engage in analytical reasoning were much less likely to demonstrate a bias than those who were primed to "go with their gut" and that

Risk

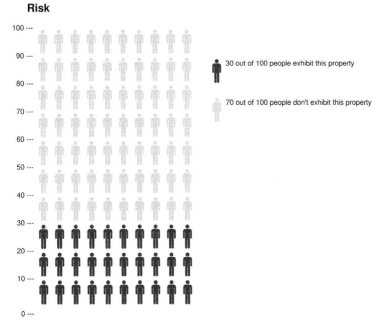

30 out of 100 people exhibit this property

70 out of 100 people don't exhibit this property

Figure 3.1 Example of a visual decision aid.

visual aids can help when framing effects coincide with low numeracy.[11,12] With regard to optimism bias – in which people tend to believe their own risk is below average – one study showed that this effect was decreased by increasing awareness about one's similarities to others at risk.[13]

When discussing such serious matters as code status, invasive procedures, and prognosis for life-threatening conditions, clinicians may not be privy to the information that should really guide these decisions: patient goals and values. As Aggarwal et al. put it, "only the individual to whom that decision relates can truly appreciate their own values and preferences and thus best interests that will be unique to them. Therefore any attempt to influence this will result in a decision that is not truly in their best interests."[14]

When it comes to discussing numbers with patients and surrogates, using de-biasing strategies, engaging them in discussions that allow for the choice that aligns best with their goals and values, and presenting information in the least complicated way possible becomes a part of the essential duty of clinicians and a core piece of shared decision-making in the intensive care unit.

References

1. N. Leiter, M. Motta, R.M. Reed, et al. Numeracy and interpretation of prognostic estimates in intracerebral hemorrhage among surrogate decision makers in the neurologic intensive care unit. *Critical Care Medicine* 2018; 46(2): 264–71.

2. A.D. Gurmankin, J. Baron, K. Armstrong. The effect of numerical statements of risk on trust and comfort with hypothetical physician risk communication. *Medical Decision Making* 2004; 24: 265–71.

3. E. Peters, J. Hibbard, P. Slovic, N. Dieckmann. Numeracy skill and the communication, comprehension, and use of risk-benefit information. *Health Affairs* 2007; 26(3): 741–8.

4. H. Friederichs, R. Birkenstein, J.C. Becker, B. Marschall, A. Weissenstein. Risk literacy assessment of general practitioners and medical students using the Berlin Numeracy Test. *BMC Family Practice* 2020; 21: 143.

5. D. Kahneman. *Thinking, Fast and Slow*. New York: Farrar, Straus, and Giroux, 2011.

6. A.R. Chapman, E. Litton, J. Chamberlain, K.M. Ho. The effect of prognostic data presentation format on perceived risk among surrogate decision makers of critically ill patients: a randomized comparative trial. *Journal of Critical Care* 2015; 30(2): 231–5.

7. S. Honeybul, G.R. Gillett, K.M. Ho, et al. Is life worth living? Decompressive craniectomy and the disability paradox. *Journal of Neurosurgery* 2016; 125: 775–8.

8. M.N. Jaffa, J.E. Podell, M. Motta. A change of course: the case for a neurorecovery clinic. *Neurocritical Care* 2020; 33(2): 610–12.

9. D.A. Zipkin, C.A. Umscheid, N.L. Keating, et al. Evidence-based risk communication: a systematic review. *Annals of Internal Medicine* 2014; 161: 270–80.

10. S. Almashat, B. Ayotte, B. Edelstein, J. Margrett. Framing effect debiasing in medical decision making. *Patient Education and Counseling* 2008; 71: 102–7.

11. A.K. Thomas, P.R. Millar. Reducing the framing effect in older and younger adults by encouraging analytic processing. *Journals of Gerontology, Series B: Psychological Sciences and Social Sciences* 2012; 67(2): 139–49.

12. R. Garcia-Retamero, M. Galesic. How to reduce the effect of framing on messages about health. *Journal of General Internal Medicine* 2010; 25(12): 1323–9.

13. P. Harris, W. Middleton, R. Joiner. The typical student as an in-group member: eliminating optimistic bias by reducing social distance. *European Journal of Social Psychology* 2000; 30: 235–53.

14. A. Aggarwal, J. Davies, R. Sullivan. 'Nudge' in the clinical consultation – An acceptable form of medical paternalism? *BMC Medical Ethics* 2014; 15: 31.

Communication Skills for Critical Care Family Meetings

Jessica McFarlin

Excellent communication is a foundation of shared decision making. As discussed throughout this book, shared decision-making is a collaborative process of (1) exchanging medical and personal information about patients' values, goals and preferences, (2) deliberation about how to apply these values to the clinical situation and (3) development of a treatment plan that reflects these values. This process is a very complex communication task. Unskilled clinicians may leave decisions largely to the discretion of surrogates without providing adequate support, and surrogates may struggle to make patient-centered decisions rather than decisions based on their own values, resulting in higher levels of post-traumatic stress disorder and depression.[1] Conversely, in a recent study of recorded family meetings regarding ICU decision-making, fewer than one-half included deliberation about how to apply a patient's values and preferences to the clinical situation.[2]

The setting for this complex task is the family meeting or the "goals of care" meeting. Data show that high-quality communication during a family meeting is difficult to achieve. After family meetings, surrogates often report inadequate understanding of diagnosis, prognosis and treatment plans.[3] Surrogates may struggle to make decisions that result in dying or changes in quality of life, even when they are consistent with a patient's values. Physicians report uncertainty about responding to emotion during meetings, endorse little time to engage in the meetings and note inadequate training to perform the skills that result in high-quality discussions.

This chapter outlines a framework for goals of care conversations during a family meeting. The purpose of the goals of care meeting is to discover the goals and values of a patient, either directly or from their surrogate. This chapter highlights the key communication skills used during these conversations to explore patient's goals, values and preferences and then make a care plan that matches these preferences with appropriate medical treatments. For the purposes of this framework, we assume that prior family meetings have taken place to establish rapport, determine surrogate decision makers,

Table 4.1. A communication framework for shared decision-making in the intensive care unit

1. Gather the clinical team for a pre-meeting.

2. Introduce everyone at the family meeting.

3. Use Ask–Tell–Ask to exchange information about the clinical condition and prognosis.

4. Respond to emotion with empathy.

5. Explain treatment options.

6. Elicit patient's goals, values and preferences.

7. Allow for deliberation about options.

8. Develop a treatment plan.

understand their decision-making preferences and deliver serious news. Table 4.1 outlines the road map of the meeting.

Of note, the skills highlighted in this framework apply to many other communication tasks in the intensive care unit (ICU), including delivering serious news and planning for end-of-life care. Not all of the tasks need to be done at once. Some families may need to reflect on and grieve over the clinical condition and prognosis before moving on to discussing values. Others may need to discuss options with extended family before developing a plan. Given this caveat, it is important to check in with family members with, "Is it OK if we talk about next steps?", to ensure it is safe to move through the framework.

4.1 Framework Steps in Detail

4.1.1 Gather the Clinical Team for a Pre-Meeting

Shared decision-making requires an accurate and consistent exchange of medical information. The meeting before the meeting with the entire clinical team is an opportunity to reach a consensus on the prognosis, explore the therapeutic options and determine the goals for the family meeting. The clinical team should include the attending physician, relevant consultants, bedside nursing and social workers. It may be overwhelming to have all of these team members present; at subsequent family meetings, the primary physician and bedside nurse should ideally always be present. Their dual presence provides uniform communications, can decrease anxiety in family members and can decrease ICU nurse and physician burnout.[4] Determine who will be leading the family meeting, keeping in mind that family satisfaction decreases when multiple attending physicians are involved in a patient's care.[5] At this time, it is also important to ensure that an interpreter is available if needed.

4.1.1.1 Meeting Location and Setup

Ensure that the meeting takes place in a private space and at a time that is scheduled with the family's needs in mind. Ideally, a conference room or designated family meeting room provides the space and seating for all involved to sit and participate comfortably. One should remain mindful of special needs, such as hearing impairment or the need to navigate wheelchairs into a space that allows everyone to participate fully. When preparing a room for the meeting, it is important that the primary physician and nurse are located in a position that allows them to both be seen and heard easily; the same should be done for the primary family spokesperson.

In many circumstances in the ICU, family meetings take place without the presence of the patient themselves. When they are able and desire to participate meaningfully in the conversation, every effort should be made to enable their participation.

When a key family member is unable to attend the meeting in person owing to timing, travel or other reasons, involving them virtually can expedite the process, prevent the spread of misinformation and allow direct questioning by the participant. In the current digital age and in light of recent visitor restriction policies secondary to coronavirus concerns, many applications exist and are readily being developed that can allow for multiperson video conferencing. In these circumstances, it is important to ensure that family participants, as well as the clinical team, are facile with the technology before the meeting, to decrease technologic frustrations that may hamper the discussion. The remaining steps of this family meeting framework should be unchanged and support the use of teleconferencing.

4.1.2 Introduce Everyone at the Family Meeting

Family can be anyone important enough, biologically related or not, to be present at a conversation with a clinician. Ensure that each family member introduces themselves and how they know the patient. Understanding these relationships can give insight into how the family makes decisions or how they support the patient and surrogates in decision-making. Each member of the medical team should also introduce themselves and their role. Surrogates do not always understand the different levels of training or roles of their healthcare team, so it is important to avoid jargon.

4.1.3 Use Ask–Tell–Ask to Exchange Information about the Clinical Condition and Prognosis

Ask–Tell–Ask is a communication strategy designed to transmit medical information based on an understanding of the patients/surrogate's comprehension of the medical situation.

4.1.3.1 The First Ask

Rather than "delivering an opening monologue" about the medical facts, the first "Ask" is an open-ended question designed to understand a family's perspective.[6]

> We know you have met a lot of doctors over the past few days. Can you help me understand everything you have been told so far about your mother's illness?

Allowing the family to share their perspective reveals how well they understand the facts and helps to determine what other information may be most helpful to the family. Listening to their perspective elicits their concerns and indicates the team is present to hear their worries. In a large family meeting, ensure that all members have an opportunity to express their understanding.

4.1.3.2 The Tell

After ensuring everyone is heard, a permission statement can signal that key information is about to be delivered.

> You all have a good understanding of this illness. Is it okay if I talk about how this affects his prognosis?

After asking the family's perspective, it is time for the Tell, succinct statements about the clinical condition and prognosis that the patient or surrogate need to understand to engage in shared decision-making. Family members want clear information about their loved one's prognosis. Audio-recorded family meetings around prognosis suggest that medical teams often do not clearly convey information about prognosis – including risk of death, ventilator dependence and functional impairments – leading to misunderstanding of prognosis.[7] The use of a headline helps families to focus on what you think the most important piece of information is. The headline encompasses both the news and how it will affect the patient.

> Your dad has serious damage to his kidneys. He will likely need dialysis for the rest of his life.
> Your husband's lung function continues to decline. He is not able to breath without the help of the ventilator, which is breathing for him.

After the headline, stop to allow the family time to think about what you have said. This information may be new. The information will be met with emotions and responding with empathy is necessary (see Section 1.3.3, The Next Ask). For other meetings, the news may be a confirmation of what they already understood and time to ask questions about prognosis, data, and certainty. Ask, "What other questions do you have?" rather than "Do you have any questions?" as you exchange information.

4.1.3.3 The Next Ask

Checking for understanding is the final Ask in the Ask–Tell–Ask tool. If a family understands the information, they can teach back the information being given. Hearing the information from the family or patient can allow for the clarification of any misconceptions, give insight in emotions and allow for further questions. The goal is not to quiz the family, but rather to ensure that the medical team achieved their goal of delivering complex medical information in a way that can be understood.

> We talked about a lot of new information. Can you explain it back to me in your own words so I can ensure I was clear in my explanation?

4.1.4 Responding to Emotion with Empathy

Receiving serious news naturally leads to an emotional reaction; in fact, emotions can be confirmation that a patient and/or family understood the information. If not attended to, emotional reactions can impede the ability to process information and consider next steps. Noticing these emotions and responding empathically is a key communication skill.[8]

Clinicians in an ICU can develop the capacity to recognize the emotional cues in a family meeting. Often the emotional cues are obvious – crying, or statements such as "shocked" or "awful." But cues can be subtle. Patients and families may express emotion with an extended silence. Cognitive questions such as, "Are you sure the test is correct?" or "There has to be something more to do," are often emotional reactions, not requests for more data. Rather than continuing to give information or disrupt the silence, acknowledge the emotion with an empathic statement. A well-placed empathic statement builds rapport, normalizes thoughts and feelings and allows exploration of goals and values.[9]

The NURSE mnemonic provides five types of empathic responses. These five skills listed in Table 4.2 can be used when an empathic opportunity arises.

4.1.5 Explain Treatment Options

The goal of the family meeting is to make major treatment decisions that reflect a patient's personal goals, values and preferences. Patients and surrogates may not be aware that there are several reasonable treatment pathways in the setting of critical illness. These pathways may include full life support, a time-limited trial of ICU care or a purely comfort-based approach to care at the end of life.[6] Families should be informed that there often are several choices and that different patients make different choices based on what matters most to them. Clinicians should provide clear information about each option without the use of jargon.

Table 4.2. NURSE mnemonic

Name	Naming the emotion shows the clinician is trying to be attuned to what is being experienced. Naming statements should be suggestive, not declarative, to avoid "telling" people how they feel	*This news seems to be a shock.*
Understand	We cannot understand the emotions others are feeling. Acknowledging this helps family feel heard and shows that you are trying to understand what they are going through.	*I can't imagine how hard it is to hear this news.*
Respect	Praising a family's ability to cope with the illness and their ability to care for their loved one is a way to show respect for their position and show empathy.	*I am really impressed by how well you all are taking care of your dad while he is here.*
Support	Statements of support can be varied depending on the trajectory of the illness. Support may be offered while awaiting test results, during time-limited trials of care or when transitioning to comfort care.	*We want to support all of you as your husband goes through this.*
Explore	Sometimes conversations may go off track or reveal information that is surprising to the physician or family. "Tell me more" statements allow the provider to further explore what the family may be attempting to understand.	*Tell me more about what is worrying you.*

4.1.6   Elicit the Patient's Goals, Values and Preferences by Highlighting Their Voice

4.1.6.1 Highlighting the Patient's Voice

To aid in shared decision-making, surrogates need the medical team to facilitate the eliciting of a patient's values and apply them to the complex medical situation. One way to focus on the values of the patient is to "highlight the patient's voice."[10] There are many questions the medical team can ask to help elicit a patient's values. Table 4.3 summarizes values commonly relevant to decisions during times of critical illness and questions that help understand the patient's values.[11]

Table 4.3. Questions that highlight the patient's voice

Has anyone in your family been through a situation like this? What did your loved one think about that?
Was it important for your loved one to live as long as possible, regardless of quality of life?
What would your loved one think about quality of life if they could not take care of daily needs or had a significant number of burdensome symptoms?
What would your family member say about their quality of life if they were unable to make their own decision?
What would your dad say is most important to him?
If your dad were sitting here and could hear what we have been saying, what would he think?

It will likely take several questions to explore what the patient values and the priority that should be given to these values. For example, a patient may value avoiding suffering, but still be willing to undergo aggressive care if it results in longevity. The purpose of eliciting the patient's values is to understand the patient's unique perception about what is meaningful to them and recommend a treatment plan.

4.1.6.2 Aligning with the Patient

As you elicit values, it is important to verbally reflect back what you hear from the patient or family to ensure alignment. An aligning statement is a summary of what you heard and a hypothesis about what it means.[12]

> It sounds like your father values taking care of his family and being a caregiver. He would want to know he tried every possible treatment to return to being able to take care of his family, but he also would not want treatment that would result in not being able to ever live at home again.

4.1.7 Allow for Deliberation about Options and Ask Permission to Make a Recommendation

4.1.7.1 Deliberation

Clinicians, patients and surrogates should actively participate in a back-and-forth discussion of the prognosis, treatment options and goals and values. This conversation is an opportunity to ensure an accurate understanding of the decision to be made, a chance to correct any misperceptions about options and ensure alignment of values. The deliberation conversation also allows time to explain why some treatments, although desired, will not work or are outside the boundaries of accepted practice. Remember that discussing treatments that will not work is essentially breaking bad news again, and NURSE statements will help facilitate these discussions. Other types of empathic statements, "I wish" and "I worry" statements, can help families to feel heard and understand when treatment options they suggest will not work.

> I wish that this treatment would help him get better too.
> I worry that waiting another week for improvement will worsen his illness.

4.1.7.2 Recommendation

As the conversation proceeds the physician should ask permission to make a recommendation based on the medical facts, the feasibility of treatments and the patient's values. Be sure to "show your work," explaining how the values of the patient connect to the recommendation being made.

> Thank you all for thinking so carefully about what is most important in this situation. Would it be OK if I gave a recommendation based on what you all have shared?
> Knowing that your loved one valued aggressive care if it might improve his chances of surviving, but also knowing he would not want treatment that would take away his independence, I recommend we proceed with a tracheostomy – but also not use CPR [cardiopulmonary resuscitation] should his cardiac function begin to decline, as this would result in not being independent in the future.

Sometimes patients/surrogates will decline a recommendation and feel that the responsibility for decision-making rests on them. Asking, "How can we best support you during this?" helps to continue to the dialogue.

4.1.8 Develop a Plan

Explaining treatment options, eliciting values and deliberating creates space to begin to develop a treatment plan via shared decision-making. If the surrogate/ family agrees with the recommendation, a concrete plan can be developed. Before the plan, always clearly repeat the decision or use a "teach back" question to ensure agreement and understanding. Avoid jargon; phrases such as "keep comfortable" or "do everything" have complex meanings to each person.

Sometimes a patient/surrogate may not agree with the recommendations. Using "tell me more" statements will help to clarify concerns about the recommendations that may be emotional or related to values. Assuring continued support of the patient during this time is essential to being able to continue with shared decision-making.

There is no one-size-fits-all path for family meetings. This framework can be a map that ensures the use of key communication skills that improve shared decision-making. When done well, shared decision-making processes may result in positive outcomes for patients and surrogates including increased knowledge, value-aligned decisions, adherence to treatment plans and decreased decisional regret.[13]

References

1. C. Gries, R. Engelberg, E. Kross, et al. Predictors of symptoms of posttraumatic stress and depression in family members after patient death in the ICU. *Chest* 2010; 137: 280–7.

2. L. Scheunemann, N. Ernecoff. P. Buddadhumaruk, et al. Clinician-family communication about patient's values and preferences in intensive care units. *JAMA Internal Medicine* 2019; 179: 676–84.

3. E. Azoulet, S. Chevret, G. Leleu, et al. Half the families of intensive care unit patients experience inadequate communication with physicians. *Critical Care Medicine* 2000; 28: 3044–9.

4. M. Kramer, C. Schmalenberg. Securing "good" nurse/physician relationships. *Nursing Management* 2003; 34: 34–8.

5. D. Johnson, M. Wilson, B. Cavanaugh, et al. Measuring the ability to meet family needs in an intensive care unit. *Critical Care Medicine* 1998; 26: 266–71.

6. A. Kon, J. Davidson, W. Morrison, et al. Shared decision making in intensive care units: an American College of Critical Care Medicine and American Thoracic Society Policy Statement. *Critical Care Medicine* 2016; 44: 188–201.

7. D. White R. Engleberg, M Wenrich, et al. Prognostication during physician-family discussions about limiting life support in intensive care units. *Critical Care Medicine* 2007; 35: 442–8.

8. A. Back, R. Arnold. Isn't there anything more you can do? When empathic statements work and when they don't. *Journal of Palliative Medicine* 2013; 16: 1429–32.

9. K. Pollack, R. Arnold, A, Jeffrey, et al. Oncologist communication about emotion during visits with patients with advanced cancer. *Journal of Clinical Oncology* 2007; 36: 5748–52.

10. J. McFarlin, J. Tuslky, A. Back, et al. A talking map for family meetings in the intensive care unit. *Journal of Clinical Outcomes Management* 2017; 24: 15–22.

11. L. Scheunemann, R. Arnold, D. White. The facilitated values history. *American Journal of Critical Care Medicine* 2012; 186: 480–6.

12. J. Childers, A. Back, J Tulsky, et al. REMAP: a framework for goals of care conversations. *Journal of Oncology Practice* 2017; 13: e844–50.

13. G. Elwyn, D. Frosch, R Thomson, et al. Shared decision making: a model for clinical practice. *Journal of General Internal Medicine* 2012; 27: 1361–7.

The Do-Not-Resuscitate Order

Timothy M. Dempsey
and Michael E. Wilson

Case

An 81-year-old woman with a history of non-alcoholic cirrhosis, refractory ascites, and previous variceal bleeding was admitted to the intensive care unit (ICU) with septic shock from spontaneous bacterial peritonitis. She arrived from the emergency department on moderate vasopressor support with norepinephrine and vasopressin. She had no family with her, but was alert enough to participate in the history being obtained. She reported that her quality of life had been gradually decreasing over the past year. She had been admitted to the ICU with septic shock and gastrointestinal bleeding two times over the past 6 months. As part of your routine ICU admission process, you approach her to discuss code status, including her preferences for cardiopulmonary resuscitation (CPR) in the case of in-hospital cardiac arrest. She asked you to do everything to help her get better – and that seeing her six grandchildren grow up is her greatest joy in life.

Even though in-hospital cardiac arrest is a relatively rare event, determining and documenting orders for CPR before the onset of cardiac arrest is important for hospitalized patients and their medical teams. Once cardiac arrest ensues, unresponsive patients are unable to participate in medical decision-making, and delays in initiating CPR may lead to poorer outcomes.[1] "Code status" conversations are dialogues between patients, surrogates, and clinicians in which preferences for CPR are ascertained. As a result of code status conversations, patients may be "full code," which entails receiving CPR should they suffer cardiac arrest, or "do-not-resuscitate" (DNR), meaning that no CPR would be performed if the patient were to suffer cardiac arrest. Other names for DNR include do-not-attempt-resuscitation or allow natural death. Decisions regarding CPR may be integrated with decisions to allow versus limit other treatments, such as the need for intubation and mechanical ventilation, hemodialysis, or vasopressor support. Sometimes, patients are unilaterally assigned a code status by the medical team (and not involved in the decision-making), although this is less common in the United States. Also, in the United States, if patient or surrogate preferences are unclear, the default code status is full code and CPR is administered.

The decision to receive CPR is often considered to be a preference-sensitive decision (meaning patients and surrogates have to be involved in the decision-making process). Shared decision-making is one recommended method to collaboratively engage patients, surrogates, and clinicians in the decision-making for preference sensitive decisions.[2] This chapter examines the incidence and outcomes of cardiac arrest and the challenges with shared decision-making for DNR, as well as methods and interventions to improve decision-making.

5.1 Incidence and Outcomes of Patients with In-Hospital Cardiac Arrest

A knowledge of the incidence and outcomes of in-hospital cardiac arrest (as well as the likelihood that an individual patient might experience such outcomes) is often, but not necessarily always, helpful to inform high-quality shared decision-making regarding code status.

5.1.1 Incidence

Although approximately 290,000 patients experience in-hospital cardiac arrest annually in the United States, the overall incidence is rare.[3] The mean cardiac arrest event rates per 1000 inpatient bed-days are estimated to be 0.58 (for all hospitalized patients), 0.34 (for ICU patients), 0.11 (for monitored ward patients), and 0.13 (for unmonitored ward patients).[4] Approximately 20% of patients with in-hospital cardiac arrest have shockable rhythms (ventricular fibrillation and pulseless ventricular tachycardia).[5]

5.1.2 Hospital Survival

Among adult patients who experience in-hospital cardiac arrest, approximately 25% survive to hospital discharge[5] according to 2017 data from the American Heart Association's Get With The Guidelines-Resuscitation registry, which includes more than 400 hospitals in the United States.[6] Although there is marked variability in hospital survival (0%–42% in published studies world-wide),[7] most larger studies in the past 10 years report survival rates of approximately 15%–25%.[8] The rate of hospital survival for patients with shockable rhythms is approximately 45%, compared with 20% for patients with nonshockable rhythms,[8] and early defibrillation is associated with improved survival.[9]

Over the past 20 years, the rate of hospital survival for patients with in-hospital cardiac arrest has increased from approximately 17% in 2000 to 25% in 2017.[5,8,10] Survival for in-hospital cardiac arrest is higher than survival for out-of-hospital cardiac arrest, where approximately 10% of adults survive to hospital discharge.[5] Several factors associated with poor prognosis include demographic elements, such as older age, non-Caucasian race, and residence in a skilled nursing facility, as well as particular comorbidities, such as renal failure, hepatic dysfunction, acute stroke, and immunodeficiencies.[11,12]

5.1.3 Long-term Survival

Although the hospital survival rate is estimated to be approximately 20% to 25%, the 1-year survival rate is only estimated to be approximately 13% according to a 2018 systematic review with more than 1 million patients.[13] Among older adults ($\geq$65 years old) in the United States who survived to hospital discharge, 59% were alive at 1 year and 50% were alive at 2 years.[14]

5.1.4 Quality of Life

Among patients who survived to hospital discharge, approximately 80% to 85% survived with an acceptable neurologic outcome at hospital discharge (Cerebral Performance Category 1 or 2; please refer Chapter 10, "Hypoxic-Ischemic Brain Injury After Cardiac Arrest")[5,14] and approximately 50% were directly discharged from the hospital to home as compared with a rehabilitation center, skilled nursing facility, hospice, or another hospital.[15] Among older adults ($\geq$65 years old) in the United States who survived to hospital discharge, 34% had not been readmitted to the hospital at 1 year, and 24% had not been readmitted to the hospital at 2 years.[14] In one study assessing the quality of life of patients after cardiac arrest, 75% of survivors were noted to be independent after hospital discharge, 17% were cognitively impaired, and 16% had depressive symptoms. These measures were worse compared with a control group of other elderly individuals, but better than that of a reference group of patients with stroke.[16]

Nearly all patients with in-hospital cardiac arrest who do not receive CPR die. Nevertheless, patients who die without CPR are often perceived to have a higher quality, less traumatic death with less pain and less distress.

5.2 Predicting the Outcome of Hospitalized Patients

For individual patients at the bedside, predicting the likelihood of survival with an acceptable quality of life in the case of in-hospital cardiac arrest is complex. The likelihood of a good outcome depends on several factors, including patient baseline characteristics, the reversibility of the cause of cardiac arrest, the ability of a hospital system to detect and treat the cause of the cardiac arrest, and the duration of resuscitation. Although published outcome data (see Section 1.2) provides baseline estimates of outcomes for large cohorts of patients, applying these estimates to individual patient situations is fraught with challenges.[17]

Prediction models have been developed to try to estimate individual patient outcomes after CPR for in-hospital cardiac arrest. One such model is The Good Outcome Following Attempted Resuscitation score (available: https://www.gofarcalc.com/). This scoring system estimates the likelihood of survival to hospital discharge with good neurologic status (Cerebral Performance Category of 1) of adult patients who receive CPR for in-hospital cardiac arrest. The likelihood of survival with a good neurologic status is based on 13 factors present before cardiac arrest.[18] The prediction model was derived and validated in a cohort of 51,240 patients with cardiac arrest in more than 400 hospitals in the United States (Get With the Guidelines-Resuscitation cohort).[18] The Good Outcome Following Attempted Resuscitation calculator was also validated externally in several populations.[19,20] It has also been adapted for use in decision aids.[21]

Hospitalized patients tend to overestimate (up to three to four times) their chances of survival in the event of in-hospital cardiac arrest,[22] possibly in part owing to media portrayals of successful recovery.[23,24]

5.3 Challenges Associated with DNR Decision-Making

No matter how many statistics patients have when trying to decide whether or not they want to be resuscitated, the decision remains a personal one, and one of the hardest patients and their families will make each hospital admission. As difficult as this choice is, the conversations preceding the decision are also challenging for physicians. This is especially true in the ICU, where there is usually no preexisting relationship between the patient and the physician and time is limited. Because of this circumstance, there are many ways this conversation can go poorly.

One of the challenges associated with deciding on DNR status is that often people who choose to be DNR are also mistakenly assumed to be patients who should not receive other treatments by members of the health-care team. Patients with a DNR order are often incorrectly considered as someone who would not want to be intubated, not want to be dialyzed, not want to be admitted to the ICU, and sometimes even not want basic treatment like antibiotics. These are distinct entities and, although the outcomes for cardiac arrest are quite poor, the outcomes for patients with respiratory failure or acute kidney injury are often better. Thus, for many people who are DNR, they may feel it is appropriate to receive a trial of other treatments, such as mechanical ventilation or hemodialysis.

Another difficulty associated with the DNR conversation in the ICU is that, even under the best of circumstances, it does not really occur at the right time or with the right person. Ideally, the conversation would happen in the outpatient setting, with an entire visit set aside for the discussion with a physician well-known to the patient, and involving both the patient and the patient's family. Unfortunately, in the ICU, this is almost never the case. This critical discussion usually occurs early in the morning in a busy unit. It almost always involves a physician who is unfamiliar to the patient and family and probably takes place within the first 10 minutes of meeting this physician. Just as important, the patient is often critically ill and not able to fully participate in the conversation. It may also take place with the most inexperienced person on the team; at academic teaching hospitals, these conversations often fall to the resident physicians. This practice can be problematic, because junior physicians may not be trained at having these difficult conversations skillfully and so may make the mistake of using medical jargon and/or not attempting to elicit the patient's decision-making preferences. It is not uncommon for junior physicians to awkwardly elicit code status by asking: "If your heart stopped, would you want us to restart it by pounding on your chest?"

In the ICU setting, patients may not be able to fully participate in the code status discussion. This circumstance leaves the decision to a surrogate decision maker, who may not know what their loved one would want in the event of a cardiac arrest. When prior planning has occurred, it may be well-informed and apply to the patient's current circumstance. When prior planning has not occurred, the surrogate may not be able to act in the "best interest" of the patient, as is expected for an appropriate surrogate decision maker.

5.4 How DNR Shared Decision-Making Can Go Well

Although it is recommended that shared decision-making be used to help patients make preference-sensitive decisions, there is no one recommended technique to use in shared decision-making for code status.[2] Different methods of shared decision-making can be used based on the different circumstances of patients.[25] Most often, a successful shared decision-making discussion involves putting the patient's overall prognosis into context with their current and previously outlined goals (if they exist). Individualized factors such as performance status, recent quality of life, prognosis for both acute and chronic issues, and pertinent and applicable national resuscitation data should be applied to allow the patient to make an educated decision.[2] Table 5.1 lists possible frameworks for engaging in shared decision-making for CPR versus no CPR.

In the first framework (option preference), clinicians would describe the options of CPR and no CPR (including the risks, benefits, alternatives, and outcomes of each option). A conversation about which option is best for the patient would then ensue. This framework assumes that a better decision will be made if the patient has more information about each option; which is not necessarily a correct assumption in all situations. Decision aids typically present decisions using this framework – and often are heavily focused on presenting the technical details of any treatment options or predictions of certain outcomes.[26] Another example of this framework is the best case/worst

Table 5.1. Possible frameworks for engaging in decision-making for CPR

Framework	Steps
1. Option preference	• Describe options.
	• Describe the benefits, harms, and outcomes of each option.
	• "Which option do you prefer?" "Which option makes the most sense to you?"
2. Agreement with a recommendation	• Formulate and share a recommendation.
	• "If your heart were to stop, I recommend we attempt to restart it with CPR. Is this all right with you?"
3. Goals of care	• Discuss diagnosis and prognosis.
	• Assess goals of care.
	• "Given this, what are your primary goals of medical care?"
	• "What is important to you when thinking about the future?"
	• Prioritize goals if needed.
	• Formulate and share the recommendation.
	• "Based on this, I recommend we attempt CPR if you heart were to stop. Is this all right with you?"
	• If needed, describe rationale for recommendation.
4. Phase of life	• Assess phase of life.
	• "What was life like for you before coming to the hospital?"
	• "What things do you have to live for?"
	• "Are you at a point in your life where you see your story continuing or do you see your story coming to a close?"
	• Assess acceptable treatment burden.
	• "How much are you willing to go through to gain more time?"
	• Formulate and share the recommendation.
	• "Based on this, I recommend we attempt CPR if your heart were to stop. Is this all right with you?"

case framework used to describe the clinical pathways associated with two different options.[27]

In the second framework, a clinician does not describe any options, but simply formulates and shares a recommended code status with the patient.

This type of decision-making may be wholly appropriate in situations where there is little ambiguity, such as a full code for a woman who just gave birth but has complications of hemorrhagic shock or for persons already on hospice care.

In the third framework, the decision of CPR versus no CPR is made only after assessing the goals of care of the patient. One example of this framework is the Serious Illness Conversation Guide.[28]

In the fourth framework, decision-making is grounded in the patients' phase of life: How much living they have to do and how much treatment burden they would be willing to undergo?

5.5 Interventions to Improve CPR Decision-Making

Several interventions have been developed and tested with a goal to improve code status conversations with hospitalized and ICU patients. A 2019 systematic review evaluated 15 randomized clinical trials of interventions in hospitalized and non-hospitalized patients to improve code status discussions.[29] Eleven trials included video interventions that often depicted simulated or real CPR. Other communication methods included a written pamphlet, scripted explanations, or conversation interview guides. Communication interventions (often compared with usual care) were associated with a lower preference for CPR (53.6% vs 38.6%; risk ratio, 0.70), a lower preference for life-sustaining treatments (risk ratio, 0.70), and improved patient knowledge of CPR (standardized mean difference, 0.55). Only one trial evaluated decisional conflict and found that a video intervention was associated with less decisional conflict compared with written information.[30] An additional, more recent, before–after pilot study of a video intervention also showed improved patient knowledge and less decisional conflict.[31]

A separate 2019 systematic review evaluated 27 decision aids on all types of life-sustaining treatments for seriously ill people near death.[26] Of these 27 decision aids, 4 decision aids specifically addressed CPR versus no CPR.[32–35] These four decision aids are available for free on the internet. To our knowledge, no large-scale studies testing their efficacy have been conducted, although the development has been described for two aids.[21,36] Of important note, routine implementation into everyday workflow remains a significant challenge.[26,37]

In addition to communication tools and decision aids, a third intervention to improve code status discussions is clinician education, especially for physicians in training.[38] One educational intervention aimed at improving communication skills involved training residents at one academic medical center on how to have these conversations through the use of an online module and workshop. The program improved the residents' comfort level with the goals of care discussions, although the study did not assess other outcomes, such as quality of discussions or changes in code status after the intervention.[39] A similar study, aimed at medical students, evaluated the use of a computer-based decision aid to help the medical students complete advanced care planning documentation with patients. This practice was compared with a standard written tool. Students who used the computer-based application had greater knowledge, more confidence in helping patients with advanced care planning, and increased satisfaction compared with the standard group. Importantly, patients were more satisfied with the computer-based program and with the students' performance on several metrics.[40]

5.6 Conclusions

Making the decision to become DNR is perhaps the most important decision patients make while admitted to the hospital. Outcomes after cardiac arrest are quite poor, although patients believe outcomes are much better than they actually are. This highlights the importance of thorough shared decision-making discussions between patients and physicians. Although many challenges exist regarding these conversations in the critical care setting, there are several methods, including providing a recommendation, that can be used to help patients make this crucial choice. Other interventions, such as decision support tools like CPR videos, have been studied and may also help to supplement physician-led discussions.

Returning to the case presented at the beginning of this chapter, the patient's physician sat down with her on admission and elicited her goals. He found that her quality of life had deteriorated to the point that she no longer enjoyed many of her favorite hobbies, such as cooking and playing with her grandchildren, because they were so difficult for her owing to her severe deconditioning. After a long discussion, her physician recommended that if her heart were to stop, she should not be resuscitated. She agreed with this recommendation and a DNR order was placed in her chart. The patient continued to receive other treatments, including vasopressor support, and ultimately improved enough to leave the hospital.

References

1. T.J. Bunch, R.D. White, B.J. Gersh, et al. Long-term outcomes of out-of-hospital cardiac arrest after successful early defibrillation. *New England Journal of Medicine*, 2003; 348(26): 2626–33.

2. A.A. Kon, J.E. Davidson, W. Morrison, M. Danis, D.B. White. Shared decision making in ICUs: an American College of Critical Care Medicine and American Thoracic Society Policy Statement. *Critical Care Medicine*, 2016; 44(1): 188–201.

3. M.J. Holmberg, C. Ross, P.S. Chan, et al. Abstract 23: incidence of adult in-hospital cardiac arrest in the United States. *Circulation*, 2018; 138(Suppl 2): A23–A23.

4. S.M. Perman, E. Stanton, J. Soar, et al. Location of in-hospital cardiac arrest in the United States: variability in event rate and outcomes. *Journal of the American Heart Association*, 2016; 5(10): e003638.

5. E.J. Benjamin, S.S. Virani, C.W. Callaway, et al. Heart disease and stroke atatistics-2018 update: a report from the American Heart Association. *Circulation*, 2018; 137 (12): e67–e492.

6. R.M. Merchant, L. Yang, L.B. Becker, et al. Incidence of treated cardiac arrest in hospitalized patients in the United States. *Critical Care Medicine*, 2011; 39(11):2 401–6.

7. C. Sandroni, J. Nolan, F. Cavallaro, M. Antonelli. In-hospital cardiac arrest: incidence, prognosis and possible measures to improve survival. *Intensive Care Medicine*, 2007; 33(2): 237–45.

8. L.W. Andersen, M.J. Holmberg, K.M. Berg, M.W. Donnino, A. Granfeldt. In-hospital cardiac arrest: a review. *JAMA* 2019; 321(12): 1200–10.

9. H.L. Bloom, I. Shukrullah, J.R. Cuellar, M.S. Lloyd, S.C. Dudley Jr., A.M. Zafari. Long-term survival after successful inhospital cardiac arrest resuscitation. *American Heart Journal*, 2007; 153(5): 831–6.

10. S. Girotra, B.K. Nallamothu, J.A. Spertus, Y. Li, H.M. Krumholz, P.S. Chan. Trends in survival after in-hospital cardiac arrest. *New England Journal of Medicine*, 2012; 367(20): 1912–20.

11. W.J. Ehlenbach, A.E. Barnato, J.R. Curtis, et al. Epidemiologic study of in-hospital cardiopulmonary resuscitation in the elderly. *New England Journal of Medicine*, 2009; 361(1): 22–31.

12. G.L. Larkin, W.S. Copes, B.H. Nathanson, W. Kaye. Pre-resuscitation factors associated with mortality in 49,130 cases of in-hospital cardiac arrest: a report from the National Registry for Cardiopulmonary Resuscitation. *Resuscitation*, 2010; 81(3): 302–11.

13. M. Schluep, B.Y. Gravesteijn, R.J. Stolker, H. Endeman, S.E. Hoeks. One-year survival after in-hospital cardiac arrest: a systematic review and meta-analysis. *Resuscitation*, 2018; 132: 90–100.

14. P.S. Chan, B.K. Nallamothu, H.M. Krumholz, et al. Long-term outcomes in elderly survivors of in-hospital cardiac arrest. *New England Journal of Medicine*, 2013; 368 (11): 1019–26.

15. M.A. Peberdy, W. Kaye, J.P. Ornato, et al. Cardiopulmonary resuscitation of adults in the hospital: a report of 14720 cardiac arrests from the National Registry of Cardiopulmonary Resuscitation. *Resuscitation*, 2003; 58(3): 297–308.

16. R. de Vos, H.C.J.M. de Haes, R. W. Koster, R.J. de Haan. Quality of survival after cardiopulmonary resuscitation. *Archives of Internal Medicine*, 1999; 159(3): 249–54.

17. J.H. Ware. The limitations of risk factors as prognostic tools. *New England Journal of Medicine*, 2006; 355(25): 2615–17.

18. M.H. Ebell, W. Jang, Y. Shen, R.G. Geocadin. Development and validation of the Good Outcome Following Attempted Resuscitation (GO-FAR) score to predict neurologically intact survival after in-hospital cardiopulmonary resuscitation. *JAMA Internal Medicine*, 2013; 173(20): 1872–8.

19. T.N. Thai, M.H. Ebell. Prospective validation of the Good Outcome Following Attempted Resuscitation (GO-FAR) score for in-hospital cardiac arrest prognosis. *Resuscitation*, 2019; 140:2–8.

20. J.B. Rubins, S.D. Kinzie, D.M. Rubins. Predicting outcomes of in-hospital cardiac arrest: retrospective US validation of the Good Outcome Following Attempted Resuscitation score. *Journal of General Internal Medicine*, 2019; 34(11): 2530–5.

21. A. Plaisance, H.O. Witteman, A. LeBlanc, et al. Development of a decision aid for cardiopulmonary resuscitation and invasive mechanical ventilation in the intensive care unit employing user-centered design and a wiki platform for rapid prototyping. *PLoS ONE*, 2018; 13(2): e0191844.

22. L.C. Kaldjian, Z.D. Erekson, T.H. Haberle, et al. Code status discussions and goals of care among hospitalised adults. *Journal of Medical Ethics*, 2009; 35(6): 338–42.

23. J.J. Van den Bulck. The impact of television fiction on public expectations of survival following inhospital cardiopulmonary resuscitation by medical professionals. *European Journal of Emergency Medicine*, 2002; 9(4): 325–9.

24. S.J. Diem, J.D. Lantos, J.A. Tulsky. Cardiopulmonary resuscitation on television. Miracles and misinformation. *New England Journal of Medicine*, 1996; 334(24): 1578–82.

25. I.G. Hargraves, V.M. Montori, J.P. Brito, et al. Purposeful SDM: a problem-based approach to caring for patients with shared decision making. *Patient Education and Counseling*, 2019; 102(10): 1786–92.

26. C.H. Saunders, K. Patel, H. Kang, G. Elwyn, K. Kirkland, M.A. Durand. Serious choices: a systematic environmental scan of decision aids and their use for seriously ill people near death. *Journal of Hospital Medicine*, 2019; 14(5): 294–302.

27. L.J. Taylor, M.J. Nabozny, N.M. Steffens, et al. A framework to improve surgeon communication in high-stakes surgical decisions: best case/worst case. *JAMA Surgery*, 2017; 152(6): 531–8.

28. R. Bernacki, M. Hutchings, J. Vick, et al. Development of the Serious Illness Care Program: a randomised controlled trial of a palliative care communication intervention. *BMJ Open*, 2015; 5(10): e009032.

29. C. Becker, L. Lecheler, S. Hochstrasser, et al. Association of communication interventions to discuss code status with patient decisions for do-not-resuscitate orders: a systematic review and meta-analysis. *JAMA Network Open*, 2019; 2(6): e195033.

30. A. El-Jawahri, L.M. Podgurski, A.F. Eichler, et al. Use of video to facilitate end-of-life discussions with patients with cancer: a randomized controlled trial. *Journal of Clinical Oncology*, 2010; 28(2): 305–310.

31. J.J. You, D. Jayaraman, M. Swinton, X. Jiang, D.K. Heyland. Supporting shared decision-making about cardiopulmonary resuscitation using a video-based decision-support intervention in a hospital setting: a multisite before-after pilot study. *CMAJ Open*, 2019; 7(4): E630–7.

32. CPR Decision Aids - Speak Up. Available: http://www.advancecareplanning.ca/resource/cpr-decision-aids/. Accessed December 29, 2019.

33. A Decision Aid to Prepare Patients and Their Families For Shared Decision-Making About Cardio-Pulmonary Resuscitation (CPR) on Vimeo. Available: https://vimeo.com/48147363. Accessed December 27, 2019.

34. Patient Decision Aid: Sharing Goals for ICU Care. Available: https://www.wikidecision.org/_media/english:final_da_english.pdf. Accessed December 27, 2019.

35. What Is CPR? Available: https://coalitionccc.org/wp-content/uploads/2014/06/cccc_cpr_web_SAMPLE.pdf. Accessed December 27, 2019.

36. C. Frank, D. Pichora, J. Suurdt, D. Heyland. Development and use of a decision aid for communication with hospitalized patients about cardiopulmonary resuscitation preference. *Patient Education and Counseling*, 2010; 79(1): 130–3.

37. S. Lund, A. Richardson, C. May. Barriers to advance care planning at the end of life: an explanatory systematic review of implementation studies. *PLoS ONE*, 2015; 10 (2): e0116629.

38. M.E. Billings, J.R. Curtis, R.A. Engelberg. Medicine residents' self-perceived competence in end-of-life care. *Academic Medicine*, 2009; 84(11): 1533–9.

39. J.K. Yuen, S.S. Mehta, J.E. Roberts, J.T. Cooke, M.C. Reid. A brief educational intervention to teach residents shared decision making in the intensive care unit. *Journal of Palliative Medicine* 2013; 16(5): 531–6.

40. M.J. Green, B.H. Levi. Teaching advance care planning to medical students with a computer-based decision aid. *Journal of Cancer Education*, 2011; 26(1): 82–91.

The Do-Not-Intubate Order

Catherine L. Auriemma
and Joshua B. Kayser

Case

Mrs. Williams is an 82-year-old woman with severe chronic obstructive pulmonary disease (COPD), hypertension, and diastolic heart failure who is admitted to the medical intensive care unit (ICU) with acute hypercapnic/hypoxemic respiratory failure necessitating rescue noninvasive bilevel positive airway pressure. She seems to be fatigued and volume overloaded on physical examination, with coarse breath sounds bilaterally. You have started diuretics and empiric treatment for a COPD exacerbation, but you worry that she may not be responding adequately to noninvasive ventilation. This is her third admission in the last 6 months. She has never required intubation, and from a brief chart review, it does not seem that intubation has been previously discussed in detail.

Respiratory failure is a common indication for admission to an ICU and can be a frequent complication of critical illness.[1] There are many different etiologies for acute respiratory failure, and the likelihood of recovery varies by underlying etiology and specific patient factors such as age, chronic comorbidities, and other acute organ failure.[2,3] While intubation and invasive mechanical ventilation can be utilized as a rescue strategy for acute respiratory failure, not all patients will find these interventions acceptable, nor is the benefit from the intervention uniform across individuals. There is substantial ethical and legal consensus that patients and their families have the right to decline life-sustaining therapies, including intubation and mechanical ventilation.[4,5]

In this chapter we will discuss the need for timely, context-specific conversations with patients and families about intubation. We will review the evidence on prognosis for patients with acute respiratory failure, suggest ways to elicit patient and family values around intubation, and describe a proposed approach to assessing the "Do-Not-Intubate" order.

6.1 The Need to Discuss Intubation Preferences in the ICU

Despite a generalized expectation of "assessing code status" for all hospitalized patients upon admission, research shows that detailed and patient-centered discussions around intubation status often do not occur, and when conversations do take place, patients are frequently not given an opportunity to ask questions and remain confused about the features of resuscitation.[6,7] Furthermore, preferences for intubation are often context-specific and can change over time.[8,9] In a study assessing patient preferences for intubation among only patients with documented code status as DNR/DNI, Jesus et al. found that over half of patients would accept intubation for a specific, hypothetical clinical situation, highlighting the need for physicians to have timely, *context-specific* conversations with patients at risk of requiring intubation.[10] In addition, it is vital to avoid conflating decisions to forgo cardiopulmonary resuscitation for cardiac arrest and mechanical ventilation for respiratory failure.[11] This is important given the different prognoses of patients with isolated respiratory failure compared to those who suffer cardiac arrest.

6.2 Epidemiology of Acute Respiratory Failure

Prognostication in acute respiratory failure is challenging as outcomes vary both by the underlying etiology of respiratory failure and by individual patient characteristics, such as age and presence of other comorbid conditions.[12] The five most common etiologies for acute respiratory failure requiring mechanical ventilation in the United States between 2001 and 2009 were pneumonia, congestive heart failure, COPD, acute respiratory distress syndrome, and sepsis.[2] In a very large, prospective cohort study of 369 ICUs from 20 different countries, the observed ICU mortality for patients requiring mechanical ventilation was 30.7%.[13] While observed ICU and hospital mortality for patients undergoing invasive mechanical ventilation has decreased over time, improvements have not been uniform across etiologies of respiratory failure.[14] Favorable trends have been observed in pneumonia and COPD, but for congestive heart failure, hospital mortality has not improved (Figure 6.1).[14]

Patient-specific factors associated with in-hospital mortality from acute respiratory failure include age, chronic comorbidities, and the presence of other acute organ failures.[15] Older age is associated with increased risk of hospital death from respiratory failure. In a prospective study of a mixed medical and surgical ICU population, hospital and 3-month mortality rates were substantially better among patients with single organ acute respiratory failure (15% and 22%, respectively) compared to patients with any other acute organ failure (41% and 47%, respectively).[3]

Certain chronic comorbidities, such as underlying cancer, are also associated with poor survival. For example, in a review of 22 studies of over 3000 cancer

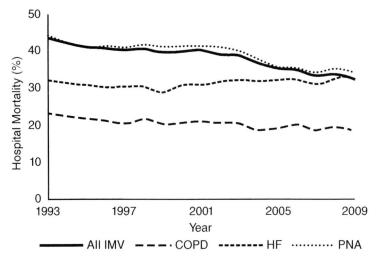

Figure 6.1 Unadjusted hospital mortality for patients receiving invasive mechanical ventilation in the United States: 1993–2009. Abbreviations: IMV – Invasive mechanical ventilation, COPD – chronic obstructive pulmonary disease, HF- heart failure, PNA – pneumonia.
Reproduced from J Crit Care, vol. 30(6), Mehta et al., Epidemiological trends in invasive mechanical ventilation in the United States: A population-based study, 1217–21, 2015, with permission from Elsevier[14]

patients experiencing respiratory failure requiring invasive mechanical ventilation, average ICU survival was 32.4% and long-term survival (ranging from two to six-months) was 10.2%.[16] Within the cancer population, the presence of chronic comorbidities and other acute organ failure, in addition to baseline performance status, are also associated with decreased survival.

6.3 Prognostication in Acute Respiratory Failure

Population-based and disease-specific epidemiologic data can be helpful, but are insufficient when considering the prognosis of an individual patient at the bedside. Modern severity of illness measures have been demonstrated to accurately estimate the risk of death in *populations* of critically ill patients, but they generally fail to predict outcomes for individuals with the certainty needed to make real-time decisions at the bedside.[17] Furthermore, survival alone is not the only outcome important to patients and their families. Physical function, cognition, mental health, health-related quality of life, and pain have all been identified as outcomes important to survivors of acute respiratory failure.[18] For many patients and their families, these functional outcomes are more important than survival alone.[19]

Incorporating likelihood of survival in decision-making for patients with acute respiratory failure is particularly challenging as the certainty of death without the intervention in question (intubation and mechanical ventilation) often approaches 100%. Rather than focusing on survival alone, patients and families may benefit from discussions with providers regarding what survival might look like. Ideally, a clinician would be able to advise the patient and family on outcomes such as the patient's expected functional status, probability of returning home, or ability to return to work, and seek to understand how these possible outcomes do or do not align with the patient's values and preferences can both help guide decision-making as well as prepare families for potentially challenging recovery periods.[20,21] Of course, these outcomes are also difficult to predict for individual patients, and preferences may change over time.[9]

6.4 Proposed Approach to the "Do-Not-Intubate" Order

Here we outline the approach to utilizing shared decision-making in the choice to undergo intubation and mechanical ventilation. This approach is adapted from models described previously.[22,23] The feasibility of completing all elements of this process may be limited by factors beyond the providers' control, such as patient severity of illness and acuity of respiratory failure, among others. However, if time and acuity allow, this process can serve as an idealized model for guiding discussions surrounding intubation status.

6.4.1 Set the Stage

This first step is often an information exchange in which the provider should discuss the patient's prognosis and the reasons for having a conversation about intubation and mechanical ventilation. The provider should offer the patient and family the opportunity to ask questions about the current clinical status as well as prognosis, answer those questions to the best of their ability, and ensure understanding of that prognosis.

6.4.2 Values Elicitation

The second step is for the clinician to elicit the patient's general values and goals for care. While previous approaches often described this step as outlining a "menu of options" and determining which interventions on that list the patient would be willing to accept, we advocate for a more holistic approach to understanding the patient's goals, values, and fears. Asking patients about their hopes and expectations for their health can be helpful. While the use of a structured conversation guide and training program to help provide clinicians with language to ask patients about their goals, values, and wishes has demonstrated promise in other health-care settings, this has yet to be studied in the

ICU.[24,25] Below, we include some suggested phrasing for value elicitation adapted to the ICU setting.

What are your most important goals for your health?

What are your biggest fears and worries about your current health?

How much are you willing to go through for the possibility of gaining more time?

Not everyone fully recovers from critical illness. What sort of recovery would be acceptable to you?

6.4.3 Description of Intervention

In the context of the patient's expressed values, the clinician can now fully explain the potential intervention under consideration – in this case, intubation and mechanical ventilation. The clinician should confirm that the patient understands the nature of intubation and mechanical ventilation, their likelihood of requiring it, and its risks, benefits, and possible outcomes. Clearly, the possible outcomes are tightly linked to the patient's overall prognosis, and in some circumstances, this can be difficult to personalize with great certainty. In general, where there is clinical uncertainty, the clinician should acknowledge it honestly.

6.4.4 Physician Recommendation

Based on the previous steps, the provider should make a recommendation about intubation and mechanical ventilation that is consistent with the patient's prognosis and goals for care. The provider should also explain the rationale underlying the treatment recommendation. Clinicians should primarily focus on the patient's values and goals when making the treatment recommendation, but should also incorporate their judgement and experience regarding which medical interventions are likely to align with the patient's values and goals. The clinician is not obligated to recommend care deemed medically inappropriate.

6.4.5 Make a Decision

As a collective unit, the patient and their family along with the clinician should make a treatment decision about intubation and mechanical ventilation. While the ultimate decision-making authority lies with the patient or patient's surrogate, patients and family members may prefer to either share that responsibility or cede it entirely to the clinician. In those circumstances, the provider should use his or her best judgement to align the decision with the values and goals elicited previously.

VALUE: 5-step Approach to Improving
Communication in ICU with Families

- V...   <u>Value</u> family statements
- A...   <u>Acknowledge</u> family emotions
- L...   <u>Listen</u> to the family
- U...   <u>Understand</u> the patient as a person
- E...   <u>Elicit</u> family questions

Figure 6.2 VALUE mnemonic for improving clinician–family communication in the ICU. Reproduced from *Chest*, vol 134(4), Curtis and White, Practical guidance for evidence-based ICU family conferences, 835–43, 2008, with permission from Elsevier.[26]

6.5 Role of Surrogates

Critically ill patients often do not possess the capacity for complex medical decision-making. Additionally, their ability to communicate with the medical team can be impeded by illness. This is particularly true in the context of acute respiratory failure, in which speaking can be both difficult and uncomfortable. In these circumstances, decision-making around intubation status, if not previously clarified, often takes place with a family member or surrogate decision maker. The same degree of care and support must be given to surrogates as we described above and in greater depth in chapter 4. If providers fail to provide adequate support to surrogates making medical decisions, surrogates can both struggle to keep the patient's preferences central to their decision-making and can experience psychological distress following the ICU experience.[26]

Unfortunately, observational data indicates that when clinicians discuss life sustaining treatment decisions with surrogates in the ICU, the patient's preference or values, particularly those around physical and cognitive functioning, are rarely elicited.[27,28] VALUE (value, acknowledge, listen, understand, and elicit) is a helpful mnemonic developed using components of clinician-family communication that have been demonstrated to increase quality of care, decrease family psychologic symptoms, or improve family ratings of communication (Figure 6.2).[29]

6.6 Evidence for Decision Aids in the ICU

Decision aids have been proposed as tools to aid in empowering the patient and their families to engage in shared decision-making and to improve the quality of medical decisions.[30] Unfortunately, there is little empiric evidence at this time to support any particular decision tool or method for supporting patients and families making decisions related to intubation status in the hospital. Experimental work has had mixed results. In a randomized clinical trial in which hospitalized patients were asked to express treatment preferences for several hypothetical clinical scenarios (including a trial of mechanical ventilation), participants were randomized either to make decisions intuitively or, with specific guidance, to deliberate on the answers and explain their choices.[31] Decision outcomes (acceptance of mechanical ventilation) and decision quality (decisional uncertainty) was similar across groups, suggesting that encouraging patients to deliberate before making choices regarding life support does not improve the decision-making process.

In another study of ICU patients already experiencing prolonged mechanical ventilation, a web-based decision aid that provided personalized prognostic estimates, explained treatment options, and interactively clarified patient values was compared to "usual care" as preparation for a family meeting.[32] Use of the decision aid did not improve prognostic concordance between clinicians and surrogates, reduce psychological distress among surrogates, or alter clinical outcomes.

6.7 Conclusions

Acute respiratory failure is a common condition seen in the ICU. The likelihood of survival in patients requiring mechanical ventilation varies by the etiology of respiratory failure, but more importantly, by the characteristics of the individual patient – with age, chronic comorbidities, and other acute organ failure predicting worse outcomes. When inviting patients and families to share in decision-making around intubation and mechanical ventilation, clinicians should first discuss the patient's prognosis and the reasons for considering intubation and mechanical ventilation. Likelihood of survival and possible functional impairments should be considered and discussed. Next, elicit the patient's general values and goals for care. Describe the intervention of intubation and mechanical ventilation. Offer a recommendation based on the overall clinical picture and the patient's expressed values and goals. And finally, seek consensus with the patient and/or surrogate to proceed with a treatment decision.

References

1. G. Smith, M. Nielsen. Criteria for admission. *BMJ*, 1999; 318(7197): 1544–7.

2. M.S. Stefan, M.S. Shieh, P.S. Pekow, et al. Epidemiology and outcomes of acute respiratory failure in the United States, 2001 to 2009: a national survey. *Journal of Hospital Medicine*, 2013; 8(2): 76–82.

3. H. Flaatten, S. Gjerde, A.B. Guttormsen, et al. Outcome after acute respiratory failure is more dependent on dysfunction in other vital organs than on the severity of the respiratory failure. *Critical Care*, 2003; 7(4): R72–7.

4. M.B. Abram, H.T. Ballantine, G.R., et al. The President's Commission for the Study of Ethical Problems in Medicine and Biomedical and Behavioural Research.

Deciding to Forego Life-Sustaining Treatment: a report on the ethical, medical, and legal issues in treatment decisions. Washington, D.C.; President's Commission for the Study of Ethical Problems in Medicine and Biomedical and Behavioural Research; 1983.

5. A. Meisel, K.L. Cerminara, T.M. Pope. *The right to die: the law of end-of-life decisionmaking.* 3rd ed. New York: Aspen Publishers; 2004.

6. J.A. Tulsky, M.A. Chesney, B. Lo. How do medical residents discuss resuscitation with patients? *Journal of General Internal Medicine,* 1995; 10(8): 436–42.

7. G.S. Fischer, J.A. Tulsky, M.R. Rose, L.A. Siminoff, R.M. Arnold. Patient knowledge and physician predictions of treatment preferences after discussion of advance directives. *Journal of General Internal Medicine,* 1998; 13(7): 447–54.

8. N. Mehta, S. Roche, E. Wong, A. Noor, K. DeCarli. Balancing patient autonomy, surrogate decision making, and physician non-maleficence when considering do-not-resuscitate orders: an ethics case analysis. *Rhode Island Medical Journal,* 2017; 100(10): 32–4.

9. C.L. Auriemma, C.A. Nguyen, R. Bronheim, et al. Stability of end-of-life preferences: a systematic review of the evidence. *JAMA Internal Medicine,* 2014; 174(7): 1085–92.

10. J.E. Jesus, M.B. Allen, G.E. Michael, et al. Preferences for resuscitation and intubation among patients with do-not-resuscitate/do-not-intubate orders. *Mayo Clinic Proceedings,* 2013; 88(7): 658–65.

11. A.C. Breu, S.J. Herzig. Differentiating DNI from DNR: combating code status conflation. *Journal of Hospital Medicine,* 2014; 9(10): 669–70.

12. S. Vasilyev, R.N. Schaap, J.D. Mortensen. Hospital survival rates of patients with acute respiratory failure in modern respiratory intensive care units: an international, multicenter, prospective survey. *Chest,* 1995; 107(4): 1083–8.

13. A. Esteban, A. Anzueto, F. Frutos, et al. Characteristics and outcomes in adult patients receiving mechanical ventilation: a 28-day international study. *JAMA,* 2002; 287(3): 345–55.

14. A.B. Mehta, S.N. Syeda, R.S. Wiener, A.J. Walkey. Epidemiological trends in invasive mechanical ventilation in the United States: a population-based study. *Journal of Critical Care,* 2015; 30(6): 1217–21.

15. C.E. Behrendt. Acute respiratory failure in the United States: incidence and 31-day survival. *Chest,* 2000; 118(4): 1100–5.

16. A.J. Huaringa, W.H. Francis. Outcome of invasive mechanical ventilation in cancer patients: intubate or not to intubate a patient with cancer. *Journal of Critical Care,* 2019; 50: 87–91.

17. W.J. Ehlenbach, C.R. Cooke. Making ICU prognostication patient centered: is there a role for dynamic information? *Critical Care Medicine,* 2013; 41(4): 1136–8.

18. V.D. Dinglas, L.N. Faraone, D.M. Needham. Understanding patient-important outcomes after critical illness: a synthesis of recent qualitative, empirical, and consensus-related studies. *Current Opinion in Critical Care*, 2018; 24: 401–9.

19. C.L. Auriemma, M.O. Harhay, K.J. Haines, et al. What matters to patients and their families during and after critical illness: a qualitative study. *American Journal of Critical Care*, 2021; 30(1): 11–20.

20. M.E. Detsky, M.O. Harhay, D.F. Bayard, et al. Discriminative accuracy of physician and nurse predictions for survival and functional outcomes 6 months after an ICU admission. *JAMA*, 2017; 317(21): 2187–2195.

21. K.J. Haines, E. Hibbert, J. McPeake, et al. Prediction models for physical, cognitive, and mental health impairments after critical illness: a systematic review and critical appraisal. *Critical Care Medicine*, 2020; 48(12): 1871–1889.

22. W.G. Anderson, R. Chase, S.Z. Pantilat, J.A. Tulsky, A.D. Auerbach. Code status discussions between attending hospitalist physicians and medical patients at hospital admission. *Journal of General Internal Medicine*, 2011; 26(4): 359–66.

23. A.A. Kon, J.E. Davidson, W. Morrison; American College of Critical Care Medicine, et al. Shared decision making in ICUs: an American College of Critical Care Medicine and American Thoracic Society Policy Statement. *Critical Care Medicine*, 2016; 44(1): 188–201.

24. J.R. Lakin, L.A. Koritsanszky, R. Cunningham, et al. A systematic intervention to improve serious Illness communication in primary care. *Health Affairs*, 2017; 36(7): 1258–64.

25. R. Bernacki, J. Paladino, B.A. Neville, et al. Effect of the serious illness care program in outpatient oncology: a cluster randomized clinical trial. *JAMA Internal Medicine*, 2019; p. 751–9.

26. C.J. Gries, R.A. Engelberg, E.K. Kross, et al. Predictors of symptoms of posttraumatic stress and depression in family members after patient death in the ICU. *Chest*, 2010; 137(2): 280–7.

27. L.P. Scheunemann, T.V. Cunningham, R.M. Arnold, P. Buddadhumaruk, D.B. White. How clinicians discuss critically ill patients' preferences and values with surrogates: an empirical analysis. *Critical Care Medicine*, 2015; 43(4): 757–64.

28. L.P. Scheunemann, N.C. Ernecoff, P. Buddadhumaruk, et al. Clinician-family communication about patients' values and preferences in intensive care units. *JAMA Internal Medicine*, 2019; 179(5): 676–84.

29. J.R. Curtis, D.B. White. Practical guidance for evidence-based ICU family conferences. *Chest*, 2008; 134(4): 835–43.

30. D. Stacey, F. Légaré, N. Col, et al. Decision aids for people facing health treatment or screening decisions. *Cochrane Database of Systematic Reviews*, 2014; 1: CD0.

31. E.B. Rubin, A.E. Buehler, E. Cooney, N.B. Gabler, A.A. Mante, S.D. Halpern. Intuitive vs deliberative approaches to making decisions about life support: a randomized clinical trial. *JAMA Network Open*, 2019; 2(1): e187851.

32. C.E. Cox, D.B. White, C.L. Hough, et al. Effects of a personalized web-based decision aid for surrogate decision makers of patients with prolonged mechanical ventilation. A randomized clinical trial. *Annals of Internal Medicine*, 2019; 170(5): 285–97.

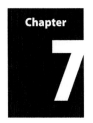

Chapter

7

Prolonged Ventilator Dependence for the Pulmonary Patient

Matthew Wilson and Philip Choi

Case

Mr. Smith is a 68-year-old man with chronic obstructive lung disease on supplemental oxygen who presented to the emergency department with influenza A and a *Staphylococcus aureus* superinfection. The patient was admitted to the intensive care unit (ICU) and underwent endotracheal intubation with mechanical ventilation for acute respiratory distress syndrome. After 10 days of appropriate antibiotics, Mr. Smith's respiratory status has significantly improved. He is now requiring minimal support from the ventilator with an FiO_2 of 40% and 5 cmH_2O of positive end-expiratory pressure. Unfortunately, he has repeatedly failed daily spontaneous breathing trials. Due to his prolonged ICU course, he is physically deconditioned and now dependent on mechanical ventilation.

7.1 Chronic Critical Illness

Respiratory failure is a common indication for admission to the ICU. The clinical context combined with shared decision-making largely determine the treatment course for respiratory failure. Advances in critical care medicine and a more protocolized approach to ICU care have allowed patients to more frequently survive the acute phase of their illness. Those patients who remain dependent on mechanical ventilation develop a condition referred to as chronic critical illness (CCI); an increasingly common trend in the modern ICU. Described by Nelson et al,[1] the hallmark feature of CCI is prolonged respiratory failure with dependence on mechanical ventilation. Patients with CCI are concomitantly affected by skin breakdown, malnutrition, anasarca, cognitive dysfunction, and profound neuromuscular weakness.[1]

CCI is particularly taxing on the United States health-care system with annual costs estimated to exceed $20 billion.[2] Patients with chronic respiratory failure often require prolonged ICU care and greater hospital lengths of stay. Given their significant comorbid conditions, these patients rarely transfer to a general medical ward. Lower nurse-to-patient ratios unique to the ICU are important for optimal pulmonary hygiene, such as frequent suctioning and help with mucus clearance. The increased need for nursing and respiratory therapists contributes to expensive hospitalizations. When patients are eventually discharged, they often require rehospitalization. As an example, patients with CCI have exceedingly high readmission rates, with an estimated 40% chance of readmission after hospital discharge.[3]

Despite surviving the initial, acute insult of a critical illness, there is notable morbidity and mortality among the CCI population. Yearly mortality among patients with CCI is estimated to be 40%–50%, which exceeds that of many malignancies.[4–6] More specifically, age and prehospital functional status are robust predictors of death after 1 year.[7] One study of long-term acute care (LTAC) patients requiring prolonged mechanical ventilation demonstrated only a 5% likelihood of being alive after 1 year if older than 75 years, or older than 65 years with poor functional status.[7]

7.2 Tracheostomy

The ICU clinician must carefully counsel patients and surrogate decision makers regarding the decision to pursue tracheostomy. Although a surgical airway may enable a patient to transfer out of the ICU, it poses significant challenges. Postoperative pain, bleeding, and surgical site infection are acute complications from a tracheostomy procedure. The long-term sequela include difficulties with speech and oral intake, fistula formation, tracheal stenosis, and the social stigmata of a chronic illness.

The ICU clinician is tasked with counseling patients or surrogate decision makers about the risks and benefits of tracheostomy. In our experience, the ICU clinician may not fully consider the complex long-term outpatient care and follow-up required for a patient with a tracheostomy. Questionnaires given to patients with a tracheostomy or their surrogate decision makers suggest more comprehensive counseling is necessary before proceeding with a surgical airway. Specifically, 80% of respondents reported receiving no information regarding services that may be needed after discharge, and 69% received no information regarding the possibility of death within 1 year.[8] Therefore, the ICU clinician should carefully explain the risks, benefits, potential complications, and overall prognosis to each patient and their family members before further considering tracheostomy placement.

There are several suggested advantages to tracheostomy. Ideally, patients can liberate from continuous sedatives that are often necessary to alleviate discomfort from the endotracheal tube. Another advantage is improved oral hygiene. The orogastric tube, commonly accompanying the intubated ICU patient, is simultaneously removed with the endotracheal tube after tracheostomy. This enables easier access for removing secretions with a suction catheter and allows the patient to cough. Last, pending improvement in the patient's respiratory status and a reduction in ventilation requirements, patients can begin working with a speech pathologist to trial a speaking valve, such as the Passy–Muir valve; the ability to communicate after a prolonged endotracheal intubation is highly valued by patients and families alike.[9]

Such benefits have, however, not been demonstrated consistently in the literature, and the ideal timing for a tracheostomy remains unclear. There have been many randomized trials and systematic reviews comparing early (defined as fewer than 10 days of endotracheal intubation) versus late (defined as more than 10 days of endotracheal intubation) tracheostomy placement. The clinical trials and systematic reviews generally demonstrate similar mortality rates, duration of mechanical ventilation, ICU length of stay, and sedation requirements between early and late tracheostomy patients.[10–13]

The largest randomized clinical trial, the TracMan trial, showed no difference in mortality, antibiotic use, or ICU length of stay in patients randomized to early versus late tracheostomy.[14] This trial highlights the lack of clear evidence for pursuing an early tracheostomy. It is our practice to individualize the timing of a tracheostomy in each patient. If prolonged mechanical ventilation is anticipated after 1 week, we recommend beginning discussions with patients or surrogate decision makers to avoid the complications related to prolonged endotracheal intubation.

7.3 Post-ICU Disposition

We consider two disposition options for Mr. Smith (our case patient), who has been diagnosed with ventilatory dependence. Outside of the ICU, patients can potentially transfer care to an LTAC, skilled nursing facility, inpatient rehabilitation center, chronic ventilator facility, or directly home. Ventilation requirements, coexisting medical problems, nursing needs, and proximity to patient's family influence disposition from the ICU.

In the first scenario, Mr. Smith can proceed with the tracheostomy and seek placement in a LTAC facility, defined by the Centers for Medicare and Medicaid Services as an acute care hospital with a mean length of stay of at least 25 days. Historically, patients would remain in an inpatient setting for the duration of their illness. The recent surge in the number and availability of LTACs have changed this paradigm of care.[15] In many ways, LTACs serve as step-down units from the ICU. LTAC physicians examine patients, make changes to help wean from the mechanical ventilation, and treat illnesses such as pneumonia with antibiotics. Patients also work with physical therapists to regain muscle mass and strength that was inevitably lost during their recent ICU admission. However, despite comprehensive medical care, patients residing in a LTAC after critical illness have a high mortality rate. These patients are medically complex with low physiologic reserve. One study noted the

1-year mortality after LTAC admission from an ICU to be as high as 52.2%.[15] The major downside to a facility-based approach is the potential distance and isolation from family. Coexisting medical problems can severely limit available LTAC placement options. The complex interplay between private medical insurance and Medicare or Medicaid may also limit LTAC availability.

Another option would be for Mr. Smith to proceed with the tracheostomy and return home. This path is now possible, given the new technology and advancements in chronic ventilation management. Returning home is oftentimes a major goal for ICU patients; the downside is the high degree of care required by family members and financial strain. Patients on mechanical ventilation require continuous care by family members, because insurance will rarely cover skilled private duty nursing. Caregivers must receive specialized training before hospital discharge for tracheostomy and ventilatory management. This intense care regimen is emotionally and physically exhausting. Caregivers of patients with CCI are at risk for depression and poor physical health.[16,17] Interestingly, caregivers of patients residing in a facility, such as LTAC, reported higher levels of depression and emotional overload compared with caregivers of patients living at home.[18]

With either approach – transfer to a facility or discharge home – patients need comprehensive medical care and rehabilitation. CCI after discharge from the ICU entails ventilator weaning, functional recovery, mental health, nutritional support, and close monitoring for development of infections.

7.4 Weaning from Mechanical Ventilation

After tracheostomy placement, clinicians and patients should continue to pursue the goal of weaning from mechanical ventilation. Ventilator weaning typically involves trials of pressure support ventilation and spontaneous breathing trials. As respiratory muscles strengthen and the patient improves clinically, the goal is to achieve adequate oxygenation and ventilation entirely without mechanical ventilation support. At that time, the clinician can consider decannulation (removal of the tracheostomy). Patients eligible for decannulation should have an intact cough and the ability to handle secretions, which should be minimal and thin. Decannulation is often achieved through progressive downsizing of the tracheostomy tube, or progressive capping trials. Many health-care institutions have inpatient decannulation protocols to ensure safety and close monitoring.

One retrospective study has demonstrated that approximately 90% of patients with chronic respiratory failure that were weaned from mechanical ventilation did so within 90 days of hospital discharge. However, unfortunately up to 25% of patients with prolonged mechanical ventilation will not wean from the ventilator by the end of the first year.[7]

7.5 Long-term Mechanical Ventilation

For those patients who continuously fail ventilation weaning trials or have a contraindication to decannulation, we briefly highlight long-term mechanical ventilation. Patients requiring long-term ventilation may reside at a specialized facility or home. Two commonly used home ventilators are the Trilogy (Respironics) and the Astral (ResMed). Among other modes, including non-invasive ventilation for patients without a tracheostomy, these ventilators can provide a standard volume or pressure control mode of invasive ventilation. These home ventilators are portable and have a rechargeable battery, thus enabling daytime and nocturnal ventilation. They are relatively lightweight and easily mounted on a wheelchair for mobility and travel. For patients residing at home in lieu of a facility, they should have a capable and trained caregiver to provide around-the-clock care.

7.6 End-of-Life Care

Patients may decline a tracheostomy in the ICU and reevaluate their treatment goals. Clinicians must elicit the values and goals of the patient. In the event the patient is unable to participate owing to an altered mental status, previous discussions or legal documents, such as a living will, may provide insight regarding the patient's views and beliefs toward end-of-life care. In goals of care discussions, the ICU physician should summarize the patient's critical care state and active medical problems. Many ICU patients have numerous consultants and, although this additional expertise can be invaluable, it may also inadvertently create confusion among family and surrogate decision makers. In accordance with the Choosing Wisely campaign, ICU clinicians should always offer a comfort-based approach to care when appropriate, such as for those with a high risk of death or severely impaired functional recovery deemed inconsistent with their desired quality of life.[19]

There are often three outcomes for patients who decide against tracheostomy placement. First, for the intubated patient with a particularly poor prognosis requiring high ventilation settings, the ICU physician may discuss compassionate extubation. These patients may experience significant air hunger, or the sensation of being able to take a full breath, after withdrawal of invasive ventilation and should be adequately premedicated with appropriate doses of opioids and anxiolytics. Medications should be titrated to achieve comfort without preventing the person from free communication if desired and able. After appropriate sedation is achieved and the endotracheal tube is removed, patients will need continuous reassessment to determine if additional escalation of these medications are indicated.

Second, there are intubated patients with prolonged respiratory failure who decide against tracheostomy, but may benefit from noninvasive ventilation after extubation. Patients who fail noninvasive therapy and have voiced

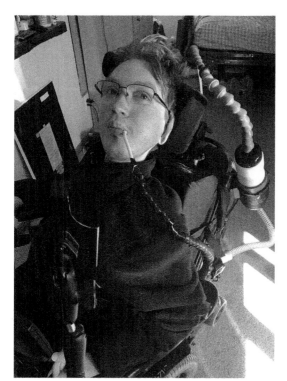

Figure 7.1 Patient using on-demand mouthpiece ventilation with a noninvasive ventilator.

their desire to avoid invasive procedures should be transitioned to a comfort-directed course of therapy. For those tolerating noninvasive ventilation, returning home may now be possible. A feature of newer home ventilators is mouthpiece ventilation. This is an open circuit form of noninvasive ventilation that allows on-demand, supported breaths without the use of a facemask (Figure 7.1). This burst of as-needed respiratory support often allows patients to complete a strenuous task or continue a conversation.[20]

Last, there are patients requiring minimal support from the ventilator who may stabilize after extubation. Although some patients may recover with mild impairment, many continue to have physical and psychological impairments that may necessitate longer term goals of care discussions. Referrals to either outpatient palliative care or home hospice may be appropriate for those patients who stabilize, but still have a high degree of symptom burden.

7.7 Conclusions

Prolonged mechanical ventilation of patients with underlying pulmonary disease may lead to a condition described as CCI. Advances in medical technology have allowed patients to survive acute critical illness, although the sequela may be a chronic state of organ dysfunction and ventilator dependence. It is imperative that ICU clinicians appropriately counsel patients or their surrogate decision makers regarding decisions to pursue tracheostomy, due to associated significant short- and long-term complications. For those patients electing tracheostomy, disposition from the ICU is typically to a LTAC or home. There have been significant advances in ventilator technology that allow for home-based care, but mortality and cost burden remain high. Last, for some patients, chronic respiratory failure provides an unacceptable quality of life. For those patients, focusing on comfort-directed care may be more appropriate.

References

1.   J.E. Nelson, C.E. Cox, A.A. Hope, S.S. Carson. Chronic critical illness. *American Journal of Respiratory and Critical Care Medicine* 2010; 182(4): 446–54.

2.   C.E. Cox, S.S. Carson, J.A. Govert, L. Chelluri, G.D. Sanders. An economic evaluation of prolonged mechanical ventilation. *Critical Care Medicine*, 2007; 35(8): 1918–27.

3.   S.L. Douglas, B.J. Daly, P.F. Brennan, N.H. Gordon, P. Uthis. Hospital readmission among long-term ventilator patients. *Chest*, 2001; 120(4): 1278–86.

4.   D.R. Gracey, J.M. Naessens, I. Krishan, H.M. Marsh. Hospital and posthospital survival in patients mechanically ventilated for more than 29 days. *Chest*, 1992; 101(1): 211–14.

5.   D.J. Scheinhorn, M.S. Hassenpflug, J.J. Votto, D.C. Chao, S.K. Epstein, G.S. Doig, et al. Post-ICU mechanical ventilation at 23 long-term care hospitals: a multicenter outcomes study. *Chest*, 2007; 131(1): 85–93.

6.   M. Engoren, C. Arslanian-Engoren, N. Fenn-Buderer. Hospital and long-term outcome after tracheostomy for respiratory failure. *Chest*, 2004; 125(1): 220–7.

7.   N.R. MacIntyre, S.K. Epstein, S. Carson, D. Scheinhorn, K. Christopher, S. Muldoon. Management of patients requiring prolonged mechanical ventilation: report of a NAMDRC consensus conference. *Chest*, 2005; 128(6): 3937–54.

8.   J.E. Nelson, A.F. Mercado, S.L. Camhi, et al. Communication about chronic critical illness. *Archives of Internal Medicine*, 2007; 167(22): 2509–15.

9.   A.M. Modrykamien. Strategies for communicating with conscious mechanically ventilated critically ill patients. *Proceedings (Baylor University. Medical Center)*, 2019; 32(4): 534–7.

10. B.N. Andriolo, R.B. Andriolo, H. Saconato, A.N. Atallah, O. Valente. Early versus late tracheostomy for critically ill patients. *Cochrane Database of Systematic Reviews*, 2015; 1: CD007271.

11. C.M. Dunham, K.J. Ransom. Assessment of early tracheostomy in trauma patients: a systematic review and meta-analysis. *American Surgeon*, 2006; 72(3): 276–81.

12. L. Meng, C. Wang, J. Li, J. Zhang. Early vs late tracheostomy in critically ill patients: a systematic review and meta-analysis. *Clinical Respiratory Journal*, 2016; 10(6): 684–92.

13. J. Griffiths, V.S. Barber, L. Morgan, J.D. Young. Systematic review and meta-analysis of studies of the timing of tracheostomy in adult patients undergoing artificial ventilation. *BMJ*, 2005; 330(7502): 1243.

14. D. Young, D.A. Harrison, B.H. Cuthbertson, K. Rowan. Effect of early vs late tracheostomy placement on survival in patients receiving mechanical ventilation: the TracMan randomized trial. *JAMA*, 2013; 309(20):2121–9.

15. J.M. Kahn, N.M. Benson, D. Appleby, S.S. Carson, T.J. Iwashyna. Long-term acute care hospital utilization after critical illness. *JAMA*, 2010; 303(22): 2253–9.

16. J.I. Cameron, L.M. Chu, A. Matte, et al. One-Year outcomes in caregivers of critically ill patients. *New England Journal of Medicine*, 2016; 374: 1831–41.

17. S.L. Douglas, B.J. Daly, C.G. Kelley, E. O'Toole, H. Montenegro. Impact of a disease management program upon caregivers of chronically critically ill patients. *Chest*, 2005; 128(6): 3925–36.

18. S.L. Douglas, B.J. Daly. Caregivers of long-term ventilator patients: physical and psychological outcomes. *Chest*, 2003; 123(4): 1073–81.

19. D.C. Angus, C.S. Deutschman, J.B. Hall, K.C. Wilson, C.L. Munro, N.S. Hill. Choosing wisely in critical care: maximizing value in the ICU. *Chest*, 2014; 146(5): 1142–4.

20. T. Pinto, M. Chatwin, P. Banfi, J.C. Winck, A. Nicolini. Mouthpiece ventilation and complementary techniques in patients with neuromuscular disease: a brief clinical review and update. *Chronic Respiratory Disease*, 2017; 14(2): 187–93.

Renal Replacement Therapy

Hassan Suleiman and Paul McCarthy

Case

A 72-year-old man is brought to the emergency department from his skilled nursing facility for shortness of breath and altered mental status. He is admitted to the medical intensive care unit (ICU) with pneumonia and septic shock. He receives appropriate antibiotics, intravenous fluids, and vasopressor therapy. He requires intubation for failure to protect his airway. By hospital day 4, his shock has resolved but he remains on the ventilator. He develops acute on chronic renal failure owing to septic acute tubular necrosis. He is anuric and grossly volume overloaded. His past medical history includes coronary artery disease, congestive heart failure, type 2 diabetes mellitus, chronic kidney disease stage III, and dementia.

Acute kidney injury (AKI) is a common occurrence in the ICU. Approximately 30% of patients admitted to the ICU will develop AKI. Of all patients admitted to the ICU, about 13% will develop AKI requiring some form of renal replacement therapy (RRT).[1,2] Dialysis can be offered via several modalities in the ICU. Continuous RRT has emerged as a popular therapy for severely critically ill patients who, in the past, may not have tolerated conventional hemodialysis. This advancement in technology has led to the ability to provide dialysis to older and sicker patients. Although the occasional patient may have previously expressed their views regarding dialysis, many families and legally authorized representatives are often faced with making the complex decision of whether to initiate dialysis without the patient's input. A discussion involving the ICU team and the nephrologist regarding expectations for mortality, renal recovery, functional status, and quality of life (QoL) on dialysis are required. The implications of developing severe AKI requiring RRT in the ICU are discussed in this chapter. Outcomes data should be used to guide discussion with patients and their decision makers.

8.1 AKI Requiring RRT: Outcomes of Renal Recovery and Mortality

AKI requiring RRT carries a high short-term risk of mortality. This serious complication is often a reflection of multiorgan dysfunction rather than a single disease process in the critically ill patient. Nevertheless, AKI is an independent risk factor for increased mortality in the ICU. A large, prospective multicenter cohort study of 17,126 patients found that the in-hospital mortality for patients with AKI requiring RRT was more than 60% compared with 15.6% for control participants matched for age, severity of illness, and treatment center.[3] A prospective cohort study found that at 1 year, complete renal recovery (an estimated glomerular filtration rate that is within 25% of the initial estimated glomerular filtration rate) occurred in fewer than one-half of the 1,292 patients enrolled (48.4%). Dialysis dependence was reported in 32.6% of patients. ICU mortality was 54.6% and increased to 72.1% at 3 years, further illustrating both high short- and long-term mortality.[4]

Despite advances in the delivery of RRT, there is no specific treatment for AKI and management remains largely supportive. The increased risk of developing chronic kidney disease and death are important prognostic implications of AKI requiring RRT.

8.2 Quality-of-Life Outcomes of AKI Requiring RRT

QoL is a vital patient-centered outcome that should be discussed with the patient or surrogate decision maker when determining whether RRT should be initiated. Many patients have strong views about life support and being kept alive by machines. It is paramount to address QoL concerns, as well as patients' and their decision maker's preconceived notions about dialysis.

A prospective cohort study compared ICU patients treated with RRT for AKI with matched patients without AKI or RRT (non–AKI-RRT) over 1 year. Patients with AKI requiring RRT alive at 1 year and 4 years were matched with non–AKI-RRT survivors from the same cohort. QoL was assessed using the EuroQoL-5D and the Short Form-36 survey before ICU admission and at 3 months, 1 year, and 4 years after ICU discharge. Of 1,953 patients, 121 had AKI requiring RRT. Long-term QoL assessed via both the EuroQoL-5D and the Short Form-36 survey were surprisingly comparable between those with AKI requiring RRT and the non–AKI-RRT group at 1 and 4 years, with no statistically significant differences detected between the groups in any subcategory of either survey. It is important to note, however, that the QoL of both patients with AKI needing RRT and non–AKI-RRT ICU survivors were lower than that of the general population.[5]

The POST-RENAL study was an extended follow-up study to obtain outcomes data on patients diagnosed with AKI who required RRT from a randomized controlled trial assessing RRT intensity. POST-RENAL used the Short Form-12 questionnaire to assess QoL in patients with AKI requiring RRT who were ICU survivors. There were 282 patients with Short Form-12 questionnaire data who were compared with 6,330 patients from the AusDiab study. POST-RENAL patients were found to have lower physical component scores (mean 40.0 vs 49.8; $p < .0001$) as well as lower mental component scores (mean 49.8 vs 53.9; $p < .0001$), which persisted after matching the participants on the basis of age, sex, and renal function.[6]

Special attention should be paid to elderly patients in nursing homes progressing to end-stage renal disease (ESRD). A 2009 study identified 3,702 nursing home residents in the United States starting dialysis. Functional status was assessed using the Minimum Dataset Activities of Daily Living scale (scores ranging from 0 to 28 assessing degree of dependence in seven activities of daily living, with high scores indicating greater difficulty). The median Minimum Dataset Activities of Daily Living score was 12 at 3 months before the initiation of dialysis and increased to 16 within the first 3 months of starting dialysis. Maintenance of baseline functional status at 3 months occurred in only 39% of patients. Furthermore, by 1 year, 58% of patients had died and functional status had been maintained in only 13% of patients.[7]

Overall, QoL data on ICU survivors requiring RRT are conflicting. It can be conferred that ICU survivors will most likely have a lower QoL than the general population. Living with chronic dialysis is at best unlikely to improve QoL and at worst can decrease physical and mental performance. Patients in nursing homes requiring long-term dialysis experience high mortality and very few maintain their baseline functional status at 1 year.

8.3 Risk of ESRD After AKI Requiring RRT

Patients and families often want to know what to expect regarding the potential long-term need for dialysis. Approximately 2%–30% of patients with AKI requiring RRT will require chronic dialysis. Preexisting chronic kidney disease and AKI severity were found to have the strongest association with incident chronic dialysis.[8] Data from the POST-RENAL study demonstrated that, of the 1,464 patients included in the original trial, only 810 patients (55%) survived to 90 days after hospital discharge. Approximately 5% were dialysis dependent at 2.6 years after discharge.[9] A separate study of ICU patients admitted after major surgery identified acute-on-chronic kidney disease as the strongest independently associated variable in progression to ESRD (incidence of 22.4 per 100 person-years and associated with a 123-fold increased risk compared with patients without AKI).[10] Individual risk factors for chronic dialysis should be assessed on a case-by-case basis with special emphasis placed on preexisting chronic kidney disease.

8.4 Shared Decision-Making for RRT

The Renal Physicians Association and American Society of Nephrology (RPA/ASN) Working Group have developed a recommendation summary based on expert consensus opinion. The nine recommendations presented in Table 8.1

Table 8.1. RPA/ASN recommendation summary

These recommendations are based on the expert consensus opinion of the RPA/ASN Working Group. They developed a priori analytic frameworks regarding decisions to withhold or withdraw dialysis in patients with acute renal failure (ARF) and ESRD. Systematic literature reviews were conducted to address prespecified questions derived from the frameworks. In most instances, the relevant evidence that was identified was contextual in nature and provided only indirect support to the recommendations. Research evidence, case and statutory law, and ethical principles were used by the Working Group to formulate its recommendations.

Recommendation No. 1: Shared Decision-Making. A patient–physician relationship that promotes shared decision-making is recommended for all patients with either ARF or ESRD. Participants in shared decision-making should involve at a minimum the patient and the physician. If a patient lacks decision-making capacity, decisions should involve the legal agent. With the patient's consent, shared decision-making may include family members or friends and other members of the renal care team.

Recommendation No. 2: Informed Consent of Refusal. Physicians should fully inform patients about their diagnosis, prognosis, and all treatment options, including (1) available dialysis modalities; (2) not starting dialysis and continuing conservative management, which should include end-of-life care; (3) a time-limited trial of dialysis; and (4) stopping dialysis and receiving end-of-life care. Choices among options should be made by patients or, if patients lack decision-making capacity, their designated legal agents. Their decisions should be informed and voluntary. The renal care team, in conjunction with the primary care physician, should ensure that the patient or legal agent understands the consequences of the decision.

Recommendation No. 3: Estimating Prognosis. To facilitate informed decisions about starting dialysis for either ARF or ESRD, discussions should occur with the patient or legal agent about life expectancy and QoL. Depending upon the circumstances (e.g., the availability of a nephrologist), a primary care physician or nephrologist who is familiar with prognostic data should conduct these discussions. These discussions should be documented and dated. All patients requiring dialysis should have their chances for survival estimated, with the realization that the ability to predict survival in the individual patient is difficult and imprecise. The estimates should be discussed with the patient or legal agent, the patient's family, and the medical team. For patients with ESRD, these discussions should occur as early as possible in the course of the patient's renal disease and continue as the renal disease progresses. For patients who experience major complications that may substantially impact survival or QoL, it is appropriate to discuss and/or reassess treatment goals, including consideration of withdrawing dialysis.

Recommendation No. 4: Conflict Resolution. A systematic approach for conflict resolution is recommended if there is disagreement regarding the benefits of dialysis between the patient or legal agent (and those supporting the patient's disagreement regarding the benefits of dialysis between the patient or legal agent (and those supporting the patient's position) and a member(s) of the renal care team. Conflicts may also occur within the renal care team or between the renal care team and other health-care providers. This approach should review the shared decision-making process for the following potential sources of conflict: (1) miscommunication or misunderstanding about prognosis, (2) intrapersonal or interpersonal issues, or (3) values. If dialysis is indicated emergently, it should be provided while pursuing conflict resolution, provided the patient or legal agent requests it.

Table 8.1. (*cont.*)

Recommendation No. 5: Advance Directives. The renal care team should attempt to obtain written advance directives from all patients on dialysis. These advance directives should be honored.

Recommendation No. 6: Withholding or Withdrawing Dialysis. It is appropriate to withhold or withdraw dialysis for patients with either ARF or ESRD in the following situations:
- Patients with decision-making capacity who, being fully informed and making voluntary choices, refuse dialysis or request that dialysis be discontinued.
- Patients who no longer possess decision-making capacity who have previously indicated refusal of dialysis in an oral or written advance directive.
- Patients who no longer possess decision-making capacity and whose properly appointed legal agents refuse dialysis or request that it be discontinued.
- Patients with irreversible, profound neurological impairment such that they lack signs of thought, sensation, purposeful behavior, and awareness of self and environment.

Recommendation No. 7: Special Patient Groups. It is reasonable to consider not initiating or withdrawing dialysis for patients with ARF or ESRD who have a terminal illness from a nonrenal cause or whose medical condition precludes the technical process of dialysis.

Recommendation No. 8: Time-Limited Trials. For patients requiring dialysis, but who have an uncertain prognosis, or for whom a consensus cannot be reached about providing dialysis, nephrologists should consider offering a time-limited trial of dialysis.

Recommendation No. 9: Palliative Care. All patients who decide to forgo dialysis or for whom such a decision is made should be treated with continued palliative care. With the patient's consent, persons with expertise in such care, such as hospice health-care professionals, should be involved in managing the medical, psychosocial, and spiritual aspects of end-of-life care for these patients. Patients should be offered the option of dying where they prefer, including at home with hospice care. Bereavement support should be offered to patients' families.

Reproduced with permission from the Renal Physicians Association[11]

should be used in conjunction with outcomes data as a framework for initiating the discussion of providing, withholding, or withdrawing dialysis in patients with severe AKI.[11]

8.5 Conclusions

The introduction of continuous RRT has revolutionized the way we care for AKI in the ICU. We are now able to provide this life-saving therapy to patients with more complex conditions and those who are sicker than ever before. When approaching the decision to initiate dialysis in the ICU, it is imperative to engage in shared decision making with the patient and/or their representative. Providing the patient and/or their decision maker prognostic information regarding mortality, functional status, and chances of renal recovery can be helpful to gauge understanding and elicit patient values. The RPA/ASN recommendations provide an excellent patient-centered framework and should be used to guide decision making. Offering a time-limited trial of dialysis should be considered in cases where it is difficult to ascertain a patient's dialysis candidacy or in patients who are unsure if they would want to continue dialysis in the long term. Palliative care can be pursued in patients who choose to forego dialysis.

References

1. E.A. Hoste, S.M. Bagshaw, R. Bellomo, et al. Epidemiology of acute kidney injury in critically ill patients: the Multinational AKI-EPI Study. *Intensive Care Medicine*, 2015; 41(8): 1411–23.

2. S. Nisula, K.M. Kaukonen, S.T. Vaara, A.M. et al. and [FINNAKI Study Group]. Incidence, risk factors and 90-day mortality of patients with acute kidney injury in Finnish intensive care units: the FINNAKI study. *Intensive Care Medicine*, 2013; 39(3): 420–8.

3. P.G. Metnitz, C.G. Krenn, H. Steltzer, et al. Effects of acute renal failure requiring renal replacement therapy on outcome in critically ill patients. *Critical Care Medicine*, 2002; 30(9): 2051–8.

4. W. De Corte, A. Dhondt, R. Vanholder, et al. Long-term outcome in ICU patients with acute kidney injury treated with renal replacement therapy: a prospective cohort study. *Critical Care*, 2016; 20(1): 256.

5. S. Oeyen, W. De Corte, D. Benoit, et al. Long-term quality of life in critically ill patients with acute kidney injury treated with renal replacement therapy: a matched cohort study. *Critical Care* 2015; 19: 289.

6. A.Y. Wang, R. Bellomo, A. Cass, et al; POST-RENAL Study Investigators and the ANZICS Clinical Trials Group. Health-related quality of life in survivors of acute kidney injury: the Prolonged Outcomes Study of the Randomized Evaluation of Normal versus Augmented Level Replacement Therapy study outcomes. *Nephrology (Carlton)*, 2015; 20(7): 492–8.

7. M.K. Tamura, K.E. Covinsky, G.M. Chertow, et al. Functional status of elderly adults before and after initiation of dialysis. *New England Journal of Medicine*, 2009; 361(16): 1539–47.

8. R. Bellomo, C. Ronco, R.L. Mehta, et al. Acute kidney injury in the ICU: from injury to recovery: Reports from the 5th Paris International Conference. *Annals of Intensive Care*, 2017; 7(1): 49.

9. M. Gallagher, A. Cass, R. Bellomo, et al; POST-RENAL Study Investigators and the ANZICS Clinical Trials Group. Long-term survival and dialysis dependency following acute kidney injury in intensive care: extended follow-up of a randomized controlled trial. *PLoS Medicine*, 2014; 11(2): e1001601.

10. V.C. Wu, T.M. Huang, C.F. Lai, et al. Acute-on-chronic kidney injury at hospital discharge is associated with long-term dialysis and mortality. *Kidney International,* 2011; 80(11): 1222–30.

11. J.H. Galla. Clinical practice guideline on shared decision-making in the appropriate initiation of and withdrawal from dialysis. The Renal Physicians Association and the American Society of Nephrology. *Journal of the American Society of Nephrology,* 2000; 11(7): 1340–2.

Chapter 9

Shared Decision-Making during Extracorporeal Membrane Oxygenation

Barnaby Lewin
and Kollengode Ramanathan

The use of extracorporeal membrane oxygenation (ECMO) supports a patient's respiratory or cardiovascular systems via an oxygenator and pump to enhance native function. Venoarterial support takes blood from a major vein and returns it to the arterial system when a patient has predominant cardiac failure. Venovenous support drains desaturated venous blood and returns it oxygenated to a major vein in cases of isolated respiratory failure. In recent years, ECMO has advanced from being simply a rescue therapy used when standard treatment modalities fail; more trained clinicians are approving it for novel indications.[1–3] Although the skills to initiate ECMO quickly have been established with structured training programs,[4] and there have been improvements to the technology to maintain extracorporeal circuits for prolonged periods to enable organ recovery or act as a bridge to further decisions on medical management, this innovative technology has presented a complex set of ethical challenges (Figure 9.1).

Although full-fledged evidence for the use of ECMO as a standard of care is still lacking, the conclusions from observational studies and randomized controlled trials do not necessarily replicate patient individuality (factors like comorbidities, insurance coverage, financial liabilities, affordability, and situations in which the individual has lost capacity to decide) during decisions surrounding the initiation, maintenance, or termination of ECMO. Clinicians and patients need to share the best available medical evidence when making decisions, thereby evoking a process of shared decision-making.[5,6] A mutually respected scenario would be ideal, where the doctor is involved in the diagnosis and establishing the prognosis, leading to recommendations on treatment while the patient or their proxies can accept or refuse the recommendation (Figure 9.1). A default shared decision-making process should include three major components: information exchange, discussion and deliberation, and eventually decision-making.[7] This chapter highlights some important aspects of shared decision-making for the management of the clinical, ethical, and patient-centered problems during ECMO initiation, maintenance, and termination.

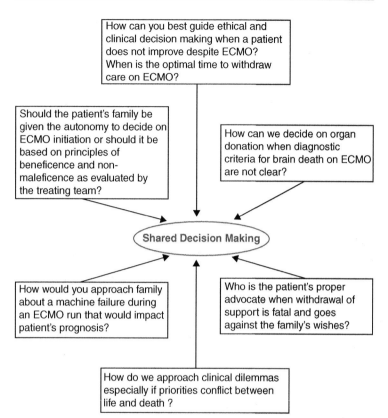

How can you best guide ethical and clinical decision making when a patient does not improve despite ECMO? When is the optimal time to withdraw care on ECMO?

Should the patient's family be given the autonomy to decide on ECMO initiation or should it be based on principles of beneficence and non-maleficence as evaluated by the treating team?

How can we decide on organ donation when diagnostic criteria for brain death on ECMO are not clear?

Shared Decision Making

How would you approach family about a machine failure during an ECMO run that would impact patient's prognosis?

Who is the patient's proper advocate when withdrawal of support is fatal and goes against the family's wishes?

How do we approach clinical dilemmas especially if priorities conflict between life and death ?

Figure 9.1 Ethical and technical aspects of patient management during ECMO that can be facilitated by shared decision-making.

9.1 Shared Decision-Making during ECMO Initiation

Case 1

A 59-year-old woman presents with a 4-week history of dry cough, with 3 days of increasing breathlessness. She has a past medical history of breast cancer 5 years back, for which she had a mastectomy and is currently undergoing hormonal therapy with tamoxifen. She presented to the emergency department with a fever and respiratory distress. Over 24 hours, she requires intubation. Her

FiO$_2$ of 0.8 yields a PaO$_2$ of 55 mmHg. Noradrenaline has escalated to 0.5 µg/kg/min. Urine output is less than 0.3 mL/kg/h. Bronchoscopy demonstrates diffuse bloody secretions. Cultures and autoantibodies have been sent. Antibiotics have been started; clotting tests are normal.

Physicians often face highly ambiguous situations such as this case when making decisions surrounding initiating ECMO. At first, we often have insufficient information to make a firm diagnosis and benefit from the viewpoint of clinical specialists as well as the results of timely investigations. In this case, the dilemma is a deteriorating patient with the need for a rapid decision for whether or not to initiate ECMO, but with the potential of underlying illness that may not be reversible.[8] In general, candidates for the initiation of ECMO include those with reversibility of illness and an improved quality of life after critical illness, as well as an absence of contraindications. These clinical decisions benefit from the input of primary team doctors who are familiar with the clinical course of the suspected illness, the ECMO insertion team, and teams that specialize in critical illness.[9]

Shared decision-making in such scenarios of ECMO initiation has its own set of challenges. Optimally, there should be rapid intervention to sustain life until there is sufficient information for more accurate diagnostics. However, this practice could lead physicians into more difficult situations where the patient is found to have an extremely poor prognosis but is stable on ECMO in the short term, and a decision to withdraw ECMO therapy would be very difficult, psychologically, for the family.[5] It should be acknowledged that this patient has a history of malignancy in the past from which she is recovering and she could be in a relative immunosuppressed state, where ECMO outcomes are poor.[10] However, the fact that she has not had a relapse after her primary surgery and that she has been tolerating her hormonal treatment would make her an eligible candidate for ECMO. There is great variability between physicians, hospitals, and health-care systems in terms of the decisions made in cases like these. A frank discussion with the patient's next of kin on the prognosis in relation to the history of malignancy would be paramount, not only in decision-making during initiation, but also during further management. A conversation with her oncology team highlighting the realistic expectations may add value to the decision-making process in this case. It is important to front-load escalation of care with family discussions, ensuring that a realistic picture has been painted; although support is being escalated, if it does not benefit the patient then it should be withdrawn to minimize suffering. It is worth noting the emotional cost families experience with an extended dying period, and the difficulty this may present to health-care staff who will be heavily invested in this patient, yet unable to achieve their aims of caring and healing.

Where a patient can express, or has previously expressed, an opinion of sound mind that they do not wish for invasive interventions during their natural illness, then a decision not to initiate therapy may be seamless.[8] The more difficult decisions surround the provision of a service in situations when a patient is no longer able to express their wishes, and the intervention may prolong life but ultimately fail, or the quality of life that is salvaged is less than would be desired. Consultation and collaboration with families to have a plan of action is critical to inform the best decision. It must be acknowledged that families consenting to ECMO initiation do so at times of high stress.[5] Families may base their decisions for expensive, resource-intensive therapies on input from friends and relatives who support the patient, insurance plans, doctors who provide treatment, or second opinions, and so on. This situation is all the more daunting in the context of ECMO initiation with ongoing cardiopulmonary resuscitation when doctors and families have limited time and opportunity to discuss and deliberate the possible pros and cons. One has to assume that truly informed consent requires time and repetition and that in this context patient proxies should be aware that no recovery of cardiopulmonary function would necessitate stopping ECMO.[5,11]

Similarly, issues of affordability and cost must be sensitively raised with the family as part of these discussions, depending on the health-care system. This point highlights one of the difficulties with shared decision-making around ECMO, given the expenses of equipment, available service, and staffing. The emphasis is more related to the ethical principle of fairness. It has been established that careful patient selection can result in improved quality adjusted life years (as found in the CESAR trial)[12]; however, this is likely to be lesser in more complex patients. It must be accepted that sophisticated treatment modalities like ECMO or cancer chemotherapy are expensive and often not 100% effective; in situations where judgements of affordability based on economic evaluation exercises would likely be challenging for families during the consenting process. In many (principlist) health-care systems the ethical tenet of justice will distribute the cost to the health-care system as a whole, whereas in semiprivatized systems, it may have economic impacts that affect families for a lifetime. Although it would be daunting not to offer ECMO to eligible patients based on financial grounds, it is necessary that health-care institutions offering ECMO have policies on initiation to deal with such ethically conflicting situations.

Collaborative care decision during extracorporeal cardiopulmonary resuscitation is also fraught with practical difficulties. The evidence for ECMO in such settings is variable between single-center, regional, and extracorporeal life support organization registries.[13,14] Discussions with families on short-term outcomes, complications, and other uncertainties, including poor neurological outcomes, can be challenging in these emergent situations. Center-specific criteria for ECMO initiation and informed consent permit appropriate patient selection, while allowing families to cope with the shock of the present situation and make an informed decision regarding the clinical teams' decision to initiate ECMO. The clinical team must revisit the need to continue or terminate ECMO at regular intervals and families need regular updating in such scenarios.[11]

9.2 Collaborative Care Decision during ECMO Maintenance

Case 2

A 45-year-old woman with a history of depression is brought into the emergency department having taken an intentional overdose of verapamil slow release (estimated at 3.8 g), diazepam (80 mg), and paracetamol (8 g). She is treated with calcium, vasopressors, and insulin–glucose–potassium therapy. She has progressive hypotension and goes into pulseless electrical activity arrest. She undergoes 25 minutes of cardiopulmonary resuscitation before the return of spontaneous circulation and is promptly initiated on venoarterial ECMO, 40 minutes after cardiac arrest.

While a patient is on ECMO, the clinical team will be presented with multiple decision points about how to optimize support. The decision points relate to the patient's clinical management with appropriate multidisciplinary teams, the need to deal with complications that are potentially reversible, changing of ECMO circuitry to support the patient optimally, and even dealing with catastrophic events related to the underlying disease process or the ECMO machine. The major ethical and patient-centered decisions in this period of time are related to complications of ECMO and progression of underlying illness. The ECMO team can use these decision points to assess the underlying clinical condition and to limit escalation.

The potential neurological recovery in the patient in Case 2 would be crucial in determining further management of ECMO. It is established that the outcomes of extracorporeal cardiopulmonary resuscitation are better than conventional cardiopulmonary resuscitation, yet the neurological outcomes are quite variable despite neuroprotective measures in the immediate resuscitation period. Although a clinical assessment of the neurological prognosis may be difficult or even limited in the presence of sedation and paralysis on ECMO, radiologic findings can assist in neuroprognostication for such patients. Evidence of hypoxic brain injury requires a detailed discussion with the neurologist, and families should be updated on the prognosis and further continuation of ECMO in such scenarios.

Complications on ECMO are not uncommon; those related to bleeding may require the stopping of anticoagulation. Although this would remain a clinical decision after weighing the risks and benefits, communication with the patient's surrogates on the pros and cons of such clinical decisions would keep the process transparent[11] and enable a future discussion of the consequences of such clinical judgements, in particular further complications like circuit thrombosis. Unforeseen complications and ECMO emergencies like pump failure can happen during ECMO runs; the team should be trained to deal with such catastrophes. It is prudent that, once the catastrophe is dealt with, full disclosure of the primary problem is highlighted in a family meeting with a discussion of the possible outcomes, including death. The family should be reassured of the hospital processes involved in reviewing such incidents, where investigations and root cause analyses would be carried out to ensure that lapses are identified, if any, and rectified appropriately.

9.3 ECMO Termination

> **Case 3**
>
> A 50-year-old woman had presented with H1N1 influenza pneumonia. She has been supported on venovenous ECMO for 6 weeks. Her acute respiratory distress syndrome has progressed through to the fibrotic phase. She failed the multiple attempts at ECMO weaning and a computed tomography scan done on day 42 shows evidence of lung fibrosis.

Exit strategies for patients on ECMO include its use as a bridge to recovery, further clinical decision-making, organ transplantation, or alternative assist devices.[8] Clinically with venovenous ECMO, a wean involves transitioning the ventilator from a "rest" to a "life-sustaining" setting, and decreasing the sweep gas on the ECMO circuit so that CO_2 is not removed and oxygen is not added to the blood. Venoarterial weaning is more complex; circuit flows are reduced and patient's intrinsic cardiac output is assessed clinically and via echocardiography. Before decannulation, it is important to discuss the implications with family, including the need to reinitiate ECMO should the patient's native function fail. Often it might be deemed inappropriate to recannulate an ECMO circuit once it has been removed because there is likely a significant physical deterioration in patient fitness after the first run of ECMO, leading to a poorer prognosis should they require repetitive runs. The family should be aware of this, and that ECMO circuit removal can mark the end of this particular phase of treatment.

The patient in Case 3 should be evaluated for lung transplantation by the appropriate teams and may be supported by ECMO until organs become available. These decisions have to be made in conjunction with the transplant and infectious disease teams; lung transplantation candidacy requires a multidisciplinary workup. Decisions regarding workup and potential outcomes should be discussed with the family by the ECMO team in conjunction with the transplant multidisciplinary team.[5]

When patients fail to achieve these end points, this intervention may end up as a "bridge to nowhere" and a transition to comfort-directed care may be in order after establishing that there is no potential for further organ recovery. This process can lead to ethical challenges that can be daunting for the healthcare team as well as the patient's relatives.[5,8] This is particularly true when cultural value is placed on the prolongation rather than the quality of life. Given that these decisions can be very difficult, it is important to have these discussions early. It may also be worth having local ethics protocols in place to prevent causing undue emotional harm. Physicians need to be cognizant that the family may take a variable amount of time with the grieving process or may not be receptive to the concept of comfort care in these circumstances at all. Please see Chapter 17 for further discussion on the role of involving palliative care consultants.

Extracorporeal donation after cardiac death is a concept that is gaining in popularity and outcomes of organ donation are found to be comparable with those done without ECMO.[15] However, ethical questions surrounding extracorporeal donation after cardiac death exist among the physician community as to whether we should consider using ECMO as a way of preserving organs for transplantation. The definitions of brain death on ECMO are subject to local institutional variability at this point in time.[16] In addition, the retrieval of organs and subsequent withdrawal of care can be emotionally challenging for staff and families, thus necessitating a collaborative decision-making approach around the diagnosis of brain death and agreement regarding the futility of care must be established before any organ retrieval may be broached. The patient's surrogates must be informed of the confounding factors that make brain death while on ECMO difficult to diagnose, including the variable pharmacokinetics of drugs as well as the impact of prolonged nonpulsatile flow on the organs.

9.4 Conclusion

The use of ECMO is growing exponentially and it is important that, with such resource intensive therapy, we continue to develop enhanced models regarding that which is possible and that which is beneficial for patients. Ambiguity remains as to which patients will benefit from this therapy and which may not.[5] Shared decision-making related to ECMO is critical, given its inherent complexity and myriad ethical challenges, and must have the agreement of critical care physicians, ECMO specialists, and other interprofessional personnel involved in the management of the precipitating illness to portray the most realistic trajectory of illness to patients and their surrogates. This summation can then inform families of expectations for the duration of the journey. Deliberations with patient surrogates must consider substitutional relational autonomy in decision-making;[17] however, appropriate emotional support and a well-established palliative and ethics consultation policy can help to alleviate the overwhelming grieving process of family surrogates during corroborative decision-making. ECMO clinicians need to be trained in specific aspects of communication skills, including forming a trusting relationship with surrogates, providing emotional support, describing other treatment options, and promoting patient preferences that eventually lead to an acceptable decision in the best interest of the patient.[18] Shared decision-making in such a context will decrease moral distress for physicians, health-care team members, patients, and families.

References

1. K. Ramanathan, C.S. Tan, P. Rycus, G. MacLaren. Extracorporeal membrane oxygenation for adult community-acquired pneumonia: outcomes and predictors of mortality. *Critical Care Medicine*, 2017; 45(5): 814–21.

2. K. Ramanathan, B. Mohanty, S. Tang, G. MacLaren. Extracorporeal therapy for amlodipine poisoning. *Journal of Artificial Organs*, 2020; 23(2): 183–6.

3. V.G. Nasr, L. Raman, R.P. Barbaro, et al. Highlights from the Extracorporeal Life Support Organization Registry: 2006-2017. *ASAIO Journal*, 2019; 65(6): 537–44.

4. B. Zakhary, K. Shekar, R. Diaz, et al. Position paper on global extracorporeal membrane oxygenation education and educational agenda for the future: a statement from the Extracorporeal Life Support Organization ECMOed Taskforce. *Critical Care Medicine*, 2020; 48(3): 406–14.

5. K. Ramanathan, M.E. Cove, M.G. Caleb, K.L. Teoh, G. Maclaren. Ethical dilemmas of adult ECMO: emerging conceptual challenges. *Journal of Cardiothoracic and Vascular Anesthesia*, 2015; 29(1): 229–33.

6. T. Bein, D. Brodie. Understanding ethical decisions for patients on extracorporeal life support. *Intensive Care Medicine*, 2017; 43(10): 1510–11.

7. A.A. Kon, J.E. Davidson, W. Morrison, M. Danis, D.B. White. Shared decision-making in intensive care units. Executive summary of the American College of Critical Care Medicine and American Thoracic Society Policy Statement. *American Journal of Respiratory and Critical Care Medicine*, 2016; 193(12): 1334–6.

8. D.C. Abrams, K. Prager, C.D. Blinderman, K.M. Burkart, D. Brodie. Ethical dilemmas encountered with the use of extracorporeal membrane oxygenation in adults. *Chest*, 2014; 145(4): 876–82.

9. J.J. Paris, M.D. Schreiber, M. Statter, R. Arensman, M. Siegler. Beyond autonomy– Physicians' refusal to use life-prolonging extracorporeal membrane oxygenation. *New England Journal of Medicine*, 1993; 329(5): 354–7.

10. M. Schmidt, A. Combes, K. Shekar. ECMO for immunosuppressed patients with acute respiratory distress syndrome: drawing a line in the sand. *Intensive Care Medicine*, 2019; 45(8): 1140–2.

11. T. Makdisi, G. Makdisi. Extra corporeal membrane oxygenation support: ethical dilemmas. *Annals of Translational Medicine*, 2017; 5(5): 112.

12. G.J. Peek, M. Mugford, R. Tiruvoipati, et al. Efficacy and economic assessment of conventional ventilatory support versus extracorporeal membrane oxygenation for severe adult respiratory failure (CESAR): a Multicentre randomised controlled trial. *Lancet*, 2009; 374(9698): 1351–63.

13. D. Stub, S. Bernard, V. Pellegrino, et al. Refractory cardiac arrest treated with mechanical CPR, hypothermia, ECMO and early reperfusion (the CHEER trial). *Resuscitation*, 2015; 86: 88–94.

14. W. Bougouin, F. Dumas, L. Lamhaut, et al. Extracorporeal cardiopulmonary resuscitation in out-of-hospital cardiac arrest: a registry study. *European Heart Journal*, 2020; 41(21): 1961–71.

15. M. Puslecki, M. Ligowski, M. Dabrowski, et al. The role of simulation to support donation after circulatory death with extracorporeal membrane oxygenation (DCD-ECMO). *Perfusion*, 2017; 32(8): 624–30.

16. C.I.S. Meadows, N.A. Barrett. U.K. National Guidelines to Diagnose Death by Neurological Criteria on Extracorporeal Membrane Oxygenation. *Critical Care Medicine*, 2020; 48(3): e266–e7.

17. N. Grignoli, V. Di Bernardo, R. Malacrida. New perspectives on substituted relational autonomy for shared decision-making in critical care. *Critical Care*, 2018; 22(1): 260.

18. A.A. Kon, J.E. Davidson, W. Morrison; American College of Critical Care M, et al. Shared decision making in ICUs: an American College of Critical Care Medicine and American Thoracic Society Policy Statement. *Critical Care Medicine*, 2016; 44(1): 188–201.

Chapter 10

Hypoxic–Ischemic Brain Injury after Cardiac Arrest

Sonya E. Zhou and Carolina B. Maciel

Case

Mr. Jones is a 65-year-old man with a past medical history of coronary artery disease who is admitted after an unwitnessed pulseless electrical activity arrest at home. He achieved return of spontaneous circulation (ROSC) in the emergency department but now remains unconscious. Upon transfer to the intensive care unit, he is intubated, sedated, and undergoing targeted temperature management (TTM) targeting 36°C. Over the next few days, sedation is discontinued as he completes TTM and controlled rewarming. Twenty-four hours after restoration of normothermia, he remains unconscious. His clinical examination is unchanged from prior: preserved pupillary and corneal reflexes bilaterally and a reflexive flexor response to painful stimuli. Continuous electroencephalography (EEG) reveals no seizures, preserved continuity, and unclear background reactivity to stimulation (Figure 10.1). Brain magnetic resonance imaging (MRI), obtained on day 4, is notable for restricted diffusion in the bilateral primary sensory cortices (Figure 10.2). Mr. Jones's family requests a meeting to discuss his chances of achieving a "meaningful recovery."

Despite numerous advances in emergency and post-arrest care, the overall rates of survival after cardiac arrest remain low.[1] A small proportion of patients recover immediately and suffer little to no neurologic dysfunction, whereas others remain unconscious for days to weeks after the restoration of forward flow. The vast majority of patients have an unclear prognosis: they lack many of the highly predictive poor outcome markers, yet they remain in an unconscious state with a likely protracted course of recovery. Thus, families and providers face a critical decision: to continue aggressive care in pursuit of a "meaningful" neurologic recovery – with the inherent risk of achieving only a profoundly disabled or vegetative state at best – or to withdraw life support. In the face of such uncertainty, neurologists and critical care specialists play a vital role in providing guidance to families. Communicating an accurate prognosis is paramount, as decisions of

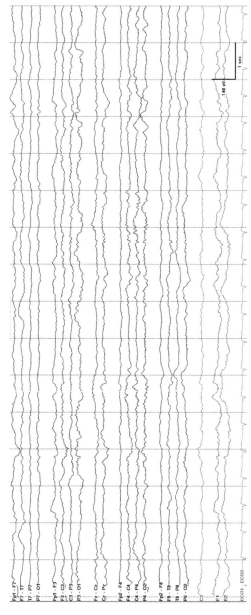

Figure 10.1 EEG with preserved continuity and unclear reactivity to stimulation.

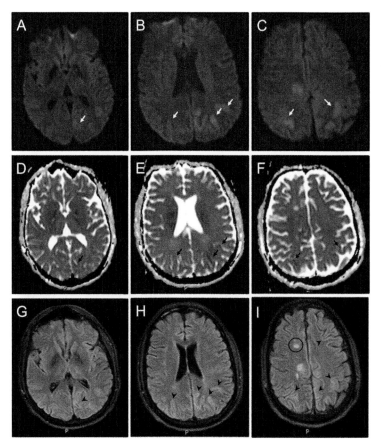

Figure 10.2 Brain MRI: hypoxic–ischemic changes in the bilateral primary sensory cortices seen on diffusion-weighted imaging (A–C; white arrows), apparent diffusion coefficient sequences (D–F; black arrows), and fluid-attenuated inversion recovery sequences (G–I; black arrowheads). Note the T2 hyperintensities in I (black circle) without associated diffusion restriction, representing findings likely unrelated to the hypoxic–ischemic injury.

continued care versus withdrawal of life-sustaining therapy (WLST) may hinge on provider–family discourse.

The goals of care discussions after cardiac arrest should contain several key elements: the estimated severity of primary and secondary brain insults, an assessment of individual cerebral resilience and the potential for recovery, and a frank conversation delineating the levels of disability and quality of life that are acceptable to individuals. In this Chapter, we discuss the usefulness of various tools used in neuroprognostication after cardiac arrest, as well as other factors that may inform shared decision-making.

10.1 Severity of Hypoxic–Ischemic Injury

Neuroprognostication begins with the collection of objective data to quantify the overall burden of hypoxic–ischemic brain injury. The etiology of the arrest, initial nonperfusing rhythm, performance of bystander cardiopulmonary resuscitation and prehospital care, and total downtime before ROSC all correlate with the severity of the initial injury from cardiac arrest.[2,3] After ROSC is achieved, other early markers of injury that reflect the postcardiac arrest syndrome include the serum lactate level[4] and its clearance rate,[5] hemodynamic instability and degree of vasopressor requirement,[6] markers of extracerebral organ damage (which commonly include myocardial dysfunction, shock liver, and kidney injury),[7] and initial EEG findings.[8]

Additionally, hypoxia and acidemia, hyperthermia, seizures, and rearrest are not infrequent. These factors set the stage for ongoing and secondary injury, especially because impaired cerebral autoregulation after ROSC leads to a mismatch between cerebral energetic demand and supply.[9,10] These additional insults can exacerbate the total damage suffered, thus challenging further the individual's physiologic resilience – currently a theoretical concept, because there are no quantifiable measures validated in practice.

10.2 Cerebral Resilience

Resilience refers to positive adaptive mechanisms after exposure to trauma or hardship. Although rooted in psychology, this concept also has relevance to neurology. In addition to the severity of injury after cardiac arrest, the patient's background characteristics also inform recovery after hypoxic–ischemic brain injury; these characteristics include age, premorbid functional state, comorbidities, prior brain injuries, and past experiences with rehabilitation. These factors interact to produce an individualized trajectory of recovery, even before the initiation of post-arrest care. Neuroimaging, obtained at any point, may help to quantify the degree of cerebral injury accrued thus far over the life course; microvascular changes, old insults, and the degree of atrophy can be visualized as surrogate markers of cerebral plasticity. Although difficult to quantify clinically, greater baseline pathology almost certainly attenuates recovery potential.

Similarly, early EEG findings and changes over time reflect both resilience and the severity of hypoxic–ischemic injury. Pathologic patterns after cardiac arrest – in particular, burst suppression in the absence of anesthetics – arise from ischemia-mediated disruptions in neurotransmission and subsequent synaptic failure.[11] Whether or not synaptic failure is reversible may depend on the degree of baseline neuronal pathology as well as the degree of acute injury. The resolution of synaptic failure and return to a continuous pattern within the first 12 hours suggests a greater recovery potential, whereas a lack of improvement within 24 hours likely represents a poorer capacity for recovery.[12]

10.3 TTM

Beginning in the early 2000s, therapeutic hypothermia after cardiac arrest quickly became standard practice, based on the results of two independent clinical trials that demonstrated improved survival and favorable outcomes in patients randomized to hypothermia, compared to those assigned to no temperature management.[13,14] Notably, neuroprognostication was not standardized in either study, and the vast majority of patients with poor outcome died during hospitalization, mainly in the setting of WLST.

After the implementation of therapeutic hypothermia, the TTM trial of 2013 randomized 939 patients with out-of-hospital arrests to a TTM goal of either 36°C or 33°C and, after a mean follow-up duration of 8.5 months, found no significant difference in all-cause mortality or favorable outcome between these groups.[15] The TTM trial raised the standards of cardiac arrest research by implementing a more rigorous and transparent methodology of neuroprognostication: all sites followed a standardized, multimodal approach.

In 2019, the HYPERION trial – the first large trial comparing hypothermia (32.5°C–33.5°C) with controlled normothermia (36.5°C–37.5°C) in non-perfusing rhythms – demonstrated a shift toward favorable neurologic survival with lower temperatures.[16] Following the example set by the TTM trial, a multimodal neuroprognostic algorithm was employed, and data on decision-making processes were collected.

Although the exact mechanism is not fully understood, the neuroprotective effect of TTM is likely driven by decreased cerebral metabolic activity, as well as decreased free radical generation and reperfusion injury; however, it remains unclear whether simply avoiding hyperthermia is the key component. Regardless, the modern era of TTM has redefined the post-cardiac arrest landscape. Because TTM may slow neuronal recovery, the natural course of global recovery is likely prolonged, and delayed clearance of confounding medications, including sedatives, may further postpone improvement. Thus, our understanding of the time course of neurologic recovery has been reset.

10.4 Outcome Measures

The Cerebral Performance Category (CPC) scale is the most widely used outcome measure after cardiac arrest. The scale (Table 10.1) ranges from

Table 10.1. CPC Scale

Cerebral Performance Categories	
CPC 1	Good cerebral performance: conscious and alert with normal functioning or only slight neurologic or psychological disability
CPC 2	Moderate cerebral disability: conscious and alert with moderate disability, independence with simple activities of daily living, and preserved ability to work in a sheltered environment
CPC 3	Severe cerebral disability: conscious with severe neurologic deficits requiring daily support
CPC 4	Coma or vegetative state
CPC 5	Death or brain death

1 to 5, wherein 1 represents a full recovery and 5 represents death. A score of 3 constitutes a state of severe neurologic disability requiring daily support despite regaining of consciousness[17]; although usually considered an unfavorable outcome, some studies do report CPC 3 as a good outcome because it reflects "awakening." Despite being widely used, the CPC scale lacks a standardized tool with which to assign scores.

The cardiac arrest literature is highly heterogeneous, and the most commonly used time points for outcomes diverge from those of other acute brain injuries, which frequently use the modified Rankin scale at 90 days as the primary outcome (see Chapter 11, "Decompressive Craniectomy for Stroke Patients"). In contrast, post-cardiac arrest neuroprognostic studies tend to employ early outcome measures such as survival to discharge or discharge CPC score, whereas therapeutic trials favor assessing mortality and neurologic outcome at 6 months or less frequently at 12 months. Understanding the timing of outcomes in these studies and applying this information to clinical practice are key aspects of neuroprognostication.

10.5 Prognostic Tools

The neurologic examination is the cornerstone for assessing prognosis after cardiac arrest. Motor response, once considered a reliable predictor, has recently been shown to carry an unacceptably high false-positive rate, regardless of TTM treatment and timing of assessment.[18,19] In contrast, absent pupillary and corneal reflexes remain robust predictors of poor outcome at 72 hours after arrest or after rewarming in TTM-treated patients. The use of a pupillometer improves inter-rater reliability,[20] and a meticulous technique with escalating noxious stimuli (from saline squirt to tactile pressure using a cotton swab applicator at the limbus) should be used to confirm absent corneal reflexes.[21]

An EEG – and whenever possible, continuous monitoring or serial short studies to capture evolution of background activity – remains another mainstay of care after cardiac arrest. Although postanoxic seizures and status epilepticus have historically been considered pathognomonic of a poor outcome, treating these conditions promptly may be beneficial,[22] and up to 50% of patients with post-arrest myoclonic status epilepticus may achieve a functional recovery.[23] However, these findings do influence the pace of recovery, and a delayed awakening is to be expected. Unreactive EEG background and persistent burst suppression are also considered malignant findings that may foreshadow a poor recovery. Nonetheless, there is significant variability in assessing reactivity, and the presence of confounders (including sedation and temperature) affects the reliability of these predictors in clinical practice.

Somatosensory evoked potentials (SSEPs) are considered one of the more reliable prognostic tools, wherein absence of N20 waves at 72 hours is considered a strong indicator of a poor outcome.[24] However, these results may be influenced by temperature and sedation and thus should be considered in conjunction with other tests.[25]

Neither a computed tomography (CT) scan nor an MRI to assess the extent of hypoxic–ischemic injury has been validated in a randomized controlled trial; however, both modalities offer potential insight into recovery. Although not sensitive, early loss of grey–white differentiation on a head CT scan is highly specific for global hypoxic–ischemic injury, with quantitative measures of ischemic changes offering greater predictive value.[26] A brain MRI, in contrast, offers greater sensitivity for ischemic changes, but at the expense of specificity.[27]

The serum neuron-specific enolase (NSE) level, a promising biomarker of neuronal injury, is not well-validated at standardized time points, and the threshold at which levels are elevated remains ill-defined. As with other tests, NSE has greater usefulness when combined with other findings,[24,28] and may offer more insight when trended serially,[29] with persistently increasing levels suggestive of ongoing secondary brain injury. More recently, serum neurofilament light chain levels have garnered interest as another biomarker, and although the data are limited currently, the initial results have demonstrated higher sensitivity and specificity for poor outcome in the first 24–48 hours compared with NSE performance.[30]

10.6 Clinical Guidelines

Several guidelines (Table 10.2) have been published to aid neurologic prognostication after cardiac arrest. The American Academy of Neurology practice parameters, released in 2006, are largely accepted to be outdated, because their recommendations are based on evidence predating the widespread

Table 10.2. Prognostication recommendations from the AAN, the ERC/ESICM, and the AHA

Guidelines for neuroprognostication after cardiac arrest	
American Academy of Neurology practice parameters	
Parameter for predicting poor outcome	**Timing**
Status myoclonus*	Day 1 after arrest
SSEPs: bilateral absence of N20 responses	Day 1–3 after arrest
Serum NSE > 33 µg/L	Day 1–3 after arrest
Absent or extensor motor response **AND** Absence of pupillary light reflexes or corneal reflexes	Day 3 after arrest

If none of the above are present, the outcome is indeterminate.

ERC/ESICM guidelines	
Parameter for predicting poor outcome	**Timing**
Absolute criterion for prognostication: Glasgow Coma Scale motor score 1–2	≥3 days after arrest
Absence of pupillary light reflexes and corneal reflexes	≥3 days after arrest
SSEPs: bilateral absence of N20 responses	≥72 hours after rewarming, or ≥24 hours after arrest if non-TTM-treated
Presence of two or more of the following: Status myoclonus (within 48 hours after arrest)	Assessed at ≥24 hours after first prognostication assessment
NSE: high** serum levels (48–72 hours after arrest)	
Burst suppression with absence of reactivity (≥72 hours after arrest or after rewarming if TTM-treated) **OR** status epilepticus (≥72 hours after arrest or after rewarming if TTM-treated)	
CT: marked reduction of the gray matter/white matter ratio or sulcal effacement (within 24 hours after arrest) **OR** MRI: diffuse ischemic changes (2–5 days after arrest)	

If the absolute criterion and/or none of the remaining parameters are fulfilled, then the outcome is indeterminate; observation and reevaluation recommended.

Table 10.2. (cont.)

Guidelines for neuroprognostication after cardiac arrest		
AHA recommendations		
Category	**Parameter and timing (when specified) for predicting poor outcome**	**Strength of recommendation**
Clinical examination	Bilateral absence of pupillary light reflex ($\geq$72 hours after arrest)	Class 2b – Level B
	Quantitative pupillometry ($\geq$72 hours after arrest)	Class 2b – Level B
	Bilateral absence of corneal reflexes ($\geq$72 hours after arrest)	Class 2b – Level B
	Status myoclonus ($\geq$72 hours after arrest)	Class 2b – Level B
	Undifferentiated myoclonic movements	Class 3: Harm – Level B
	Absent or extensor motor response in upper extremities	Class 3: Harm – Level B
EEG	Persistent status epilepticus ($\geq$72 hours after arrest)	Class 2b – Level B
	Burst suppression ($\geq$72 hours after arrest)	Class 2b – Level B
	Absence of EEG reactivity (within 72 hours after arrest)	Class 3: No benefit – Level B
SSEPs	Bilateral absence of N20 waves ($\geq$24 hours after arrest)	Class 2b – Level B
Neuroimaging	CT: reduced gray-white ratio	Class 2b – Level B
	MRI: extensive areas of restricted diffusion (days 2–7)	Class 2b – Level B
	MRI: extensive areas of reduced apparent diffusion coefficient (days 2–7)	Class 2b – Level B
Biomarkers	NSE: high** serum values (within 72 hours after arrest)	Class 2b – Level B
	S100 calcium-binding protein, Tau, neurofilament light chain, glial fibrillary acidic protein	Class 2b – Level C – usefulness uncertain

* Clinical diagnosis; no definition provided.
** No NSE threshold recommended.

implementation of TTM.[31] In 2014, the European Resuscitation Council and European Society of Intensive Care Medicine (ERC/ESICM) published their own evidence-based, multimodal algorithm[24] that reaffirms the negative predictive value of absent pupillary and corneal reflexes on days 3–5, as well as that of bilaterally absent N20 waves on SSEPs. Both predict a "very likely" poor outcome with a false-positive rate of less than 5%. In the absence of these findings, an elevated NSE, prolonged status myoclonus, malignant EEG patterns, and radiologic evidence of hypoxic–ischemic injury may predict poor recovery, particularly when found in conjunction with one another. Notably, the ERC/ESICM guidelines apply only to patients with an absent or extensor motor response at the time of prognostication.

In the recently updated 2020 guidelines, the American Heart Association (AHA) presents its own multimodal approach to prognostication, employing features of the neurologic examination as well as neuroimaging studies, EEG, SSEPs, and serum NSE testing.[32] However, none of these individual tests boasts a strong class of recommendation or level of evidence rating for predicting a poor neurologic outcome, with the AHA acknowledging that the overall quality of evidence in the literature is low due to the inherent biases in most studies as well as limited generalizability. Thus, although the AHA assesses the strength of evidence for various tests in isolation, each test is recommended for use in combination with other findings, and no specific combination of findings is presented as a reliable predictor of a poor neurologic outcome.

In a 2019 single-center, retrospective study of 226 patients comparing the performances of the guidelines detailed in Table 10.2 (though, of note, the earlier AHA guidelines from 2015 were used), the ERC/ESICM algorithm maintained the highest specificity (false-positive rate of 0%) for predicting a poor outcome. However, its sensitivity for poor outcome was less than 30%.[33]

10.7 Timing of Prognostication

The cardiac arrest literature to date is marred by the bias of a self-fulfilling prophecy,[34] in which test results used to predict an unfavorable prognosis dictate the decision for WLST, thus inevitably confirming the predicted outcome. In these situations, perhaps the patient may have had a good recovery, despite the initial findings, had supportive care been maintained. Although unnecessarily prolonging care in the setting of an inevitably poor outcome is undesirable, so too is premature WLST in a patient who will achieve a good outcome. Recently, there have been reports of patients demonstrating delayed awakening and recovery, beyond the first few days – and sometimes weeks – after arrest.[35–37]

When the prognosis remains uncertain, providers must resist the temptation to convey a definitive outcome, and instead may favor additional time to observe for changes or improvements. The pace of neurologic recovery is highly variable, and time to awakening can be influenced by factors including organ (e.g., renal or liver) dysfunction, use of TTM with lower target temperatures, sedation, and postanoxic status epilepticus. The current recommendation is to delay prognostication for at least 72 hours after rewarming, or 72 hours after arrest if TTM has not been employed; but even then, in the setting of uncertainty or confounders, further delay is likely warranted.[24,38]

10.8 Balancing Empirical Data with Patient Values

Even before the collection of prognostic data, the details of the arrest, the patient's background and cerebral resilience, the extent of secondary injury, and personal preferences all frame the individual patient experience. From there, clinical findings only further mold the prognosis. As in any encounter, shared decisions must account for a patient's unique circumstances. The guidelines are not meant to dictate; rather, they provide a reasonable expectation of recovery based on the average patient, with the caveat that this average patient is in fact derived from an amalgam of widely varied and unique characteristics and circumstances. Nonetheless, these guidelines offer a tangible, evidence-based expectation that can be conveyed to families.

Beyond the predicted outcome, the journey of recovery also warrants candid and detailed discussion with families. Recovery may be slow and drawn out, with a range of neurologic and functional limitations, and the time course to achieve the best expected outcome adds further uncertainty; few studies have assessed recovery beyond the first 6–12 months.

Finally, prognostication is not a singular event, nor is there a single time point at which it should occur. Rather, accurate prognostication stems from a collection of data at various times, all of which interact to produce a depiction of expected recovery. Moreover, it must be remembered that the foundation of evidence that underlies the aforementioned guidelines is based on arbitrary definitions of "good" versus "bad" outcomes. Yet, ultimately, how one defines a good outcome is subjective; a CPC score of 3 may be acceptable for one patient but not for another. Of utmost importance during these shared decision-making processes is to gauge what constitutes a satisfactory quality of life to the individual patient. Providers must also be conscious of their own biases when assessing prognosis.

10.9 Conclusions

After survival from cardiac arrest, the range of outcomes varies widely, particularly for those who remain unconscious in the aftermath. Providers and families may feel pressured to make prompt decisions on the continuation versus the withdrawal of care; however, the usefulness of various prognostic tests is highly sensitive to time, and when in doubt, the optimal strategy may be to wait. Caution should be applied when conveying expected outcomes to families, as these expectations are often uncertain and fluid. Finally, prognostic assessments should consider the characteristics of the individual patient – not only the extent of damage suffered from the arrest but also the patient's own background and prior level of functioning – and all shared decisions must account for the patient's core values and beliefs around a meaningful quality of life.

References

1. E.J. Benjamin, P. Muntner, A. Alonso, et al. Heart disease and stroke statistics-2019 update: a Report From the American Heart Association. *Circulation*, 2019; 139(10): e56–e528.

2. Y. Xiong, H. Zhan, Y. Lu, et al. Out-of-hospital cardiac arrest without return of spontaneous circulation in the field: Who are the survivors? *Resuscitation*, 2017; 112: 28–33.

3. S. Rajan, F. Folke, S.M. Hansen, et al. Incidence and survival outcome according to heart rhythm during resuscitation attempt in out-of-hospital cardiac arrest patients with presumed cardiac etiology. *Resuscitation*, 2017; 114: 157–63.

4. C.H. Wang, C.H. Huang, W.T. Chang, et al. Monitoring of serum lactate level during cardiopulmonary resuscitation in adult in-hospital cardiac arrest. *Critical Care*, 2015; 19: 344.

5. T.R. Lee, M.J. Kang, W.C. Cha, et al. Better lactate clearance associated with good neurologic outcome in survivors who treated with therapeutic hypothermia after out-of-hospital cardiac arrest. *Critical Care*, 2013; 17(5): R260.

6. C.H. Huang, M.S. Tsai, H.N. Ong, W. et al. Association of hemodynamic variables with in-hospital mortality and favorable neurological outcomes in post-cardiac arrest care with targeted temperature management. *Resuscitation*, 2017; 120: 146–52.

7. L. Nobile, F.S. Taccone, T. Szakmany, et al. The impact of extracerebral organ failure on outcome of patients after cardiac arrest: an observational study from the ICON database. *Critical Care*, 2016; 20(1): 368.

8. A. O. Rossetti, E. Carrera, M. Oddo. Early EEG correlates of neuronal injury after brain anoxia. *Neurology*, 2012; 78(11): 796–802.

9. J.M. van den Brule, E. Vinke, L.M. van Loon, et al. Middle cerebral artery flow, the critical closing pressure, and the optimal mean arterial pressure in comatose cardiac arrest survivors: an observational study. *Resuscitation*, 2017; 110: 85–9.

10. V. Lemiale, O. Huet, B. Vigue, et al. Changes in cerebral blood flow and oxygen extraction during post-resuscitation syndrome. *Resuscitation*, 2008; 76(1): 17–24.

11. M.J. van Putten, J. Hofmeijer. Generalized periodic discharges: pathophysiology and clinical considerations. *Epilepsy & Behavior: E&B* 2015; 49: 228–33.

12. M.J. van Putten, J. Hofmeijer. EEG monitoring in cerebral ischemia: basic concepts and clinical applications. *Journal of Clinical Neurophysiology*, 2016; 33(3): 203–10.

13. S.A. Bernard, T.W. Gray, M.D. Buist, et al. Treatment of comatose survivors of out-of-hospital cardiac arrest with induced hypothermia. *New England Journal of Medicine*, 2002; 346(8): 557–63.

14. Hypothermia after Cardiac Arrest Study Group. Mild therapeutic hypothermia to improve the neurologic outcome after cardiac arrest. *New England Journal of Medicine*, 2002; 346(8): 549–56.

15. N. Nielsen, J. Wetterslev, T. Cronberg, et al. Targeted temperature management at 33 degrees C versus 36 degrees C after cardiac arrest. *New England Journal of Medicine*, 2013; 369(23): 2197–206.

16. J.B. Lascarrou, H. Merdji, A. Le Gouge, et al. Targeted temperature management for cardiac arrest with nonshockable rhythm. *New England Journal of Medicine*,. 2019; 381: 2327–37.

17. P. Safar. Resuscitation after brain ischemia. *Brain Failure and Resuscitation*, 1981; 155: 184.

18. C. Sandroni, F. Cavallaro, C.W. Callaway, et al. Predictors of poor neurological outcome in adult comatose survivors of cardiac arrest: a systematic review and meta-analysis. Part 2: Patients treated with therapeutic hypothermia. *Resuscitation*, 2013; 84(10): 1324–38.

19. C. Sandroni, F. Cavallaro, C.W. Callaway, et al. Predictors of poor neurological outcome in adult comatose survivors of cardiac arrest: A systematic review and meta-analysis. Part 1: Patients not treated with therapeutic hypothermia. *Resuscitation*, 2013; 84(10): 1310–23.

20. M. Oddo, C. Sandroni, G. Citerio, et al. Quantitative versus standard pupillary light reflex for early prognostication in comatose cardiac arrest patients: an international prospective multicenter double-blinded study. *Intensive Care Medicine*, 2018; 44 (12): 2102–11.

21. C.B. Maciel, T.S. Youn, M.M. Barden, et al. Corneal reflex testing in the evaluation of a comatose patient: an ode to precise semiology and exmination skills. *Neurocritical Care*, 2020; 33(2): 399–404.

22. S. Beretta, A. Coppo, E. Bianchi, et al. Neurologic outcome of postanoxic refractory status epilepticus after aggressive treatment. *Neurology*, 2018; 91(23): e2153–e62.

23. J. Elmer, J.C. Rittenberger, J. Faro, et al. Clinically distinct electroencephalographic phenotypes of early myoclonus after cardiac arrest. *Annals of Neurology*, 2016; 80(2): 175–84.

24. J.P. Nolan, J. Soar, A. Cariou, et al. European Resuscitation Council and European Society of Intensive Care Medicine 2015 guidelines for post-resuscitation care. *Intensive Care Medicine*, 2015; 41(12): 2039–56.

25. C.B. Maciel, A.O. Morawo, C.Y. Tsao, et al. SSEP in Therapeutic Hypothermia Era. *Journal of Clinical Neurophysiology*, 2017; 34(5): 469–75.

26. C. Cristia, M.L. Ho, S. Levy, et al. The association between a quantitative computed tomography (CT) measurement of cerebral edema and outcomes in post-cardiac arrest-a validation study. *Resuscitation*, 2014; 85(10): 1348–53.

27. D. Greer, P. Scripko, J. Bartscher, et al. Clinical MRI interpretation for outcome prediction in cardiac arrest. *Neurocritical Care*, 2012; 17(2): 240–4.

28. M. Oddo, A.O. Rossetti. Early multimodal outcome prediction after cardiac arrest in patients treated with hypothermia. *Critical Care Medicine*, 2014; 42(6): 1340–7.

29. S. Wiberg, C. Hassager, P. Stammet, et al. Single versus serial measurements of neuron-specific enolase and prediction of poor neurological outcome in persistently unconscious patients after out-of-hospital cardiac arrest - A TTM-Trial Substudy. *PLoS ONE*, 2017; 12(1): e0168894.

30. M. Moseby-Knappe, N. Mattsson, N. Nielsen, et al. Serum neurofilament light chain for prognosis of outcome after cardiac arrest. *JAMA Neurology*, 2019; 76(1): 64–71.

31. E.F. Wijdicks, A. Hijdra, G.B. Young, et al. Quality Standards Subcommittee of the American Academy of N. Practice parameter: prediction of outcome in comatose survivors after cardiopulmonary resuscitation (an evidence-based review): report of the Quality Standards Subcommittee of the American Academy of Neurology. *Neurology*, 2006; 67(2): 203–10.

32. A.R. Panchal, J.A. Bartos, J.G. Cabañas, et al. Part 3: Adult Basic and Advanced Life Support: 2020 American Heart Association Guidelines for Cardiopulmonary Resuscitation and Emergency Cardiovascular Care. *Circulation*, 2020; 142(16 Suppl 2): S366–468.

33. S.E. Zhou, C.B. Maciel, C.H. Ormseth, et al. Distinct predictive values of current neuroprognostic guidelines in post-cardiac arrest patients. *Resuscitation*, 2019; 139: 343–50.

34. R.G. Geocadin, M.A. Peberdy, R.M. Lazar. Poor survival after cardiac arrest resuscitation: a self-fulfilling prophecy or biologic destiny?. *Critical Care Medicine*, 2012; 40(3): 979–80.

35. A.V. Grossestreuer, B.S. Abella, M. Leary, et al. Time to awakening and neurologic outcome in therapeutic hypothermia-treated cardiac arrest patients. *Resuscitation*, 2013; 84(12): 1741–6.

36. K. Zanyk-McLean, K.N. Sawyer, R. Paternoster, et al. Time to awakening is often delayed in patients who receive targeted temperature management after cardiac arrest. *Therapeutic Hypothermia and Temperature Management*, 2017; 7(2): 95–100.

37. D.M. Greer. Unexpected good recovery in a comatose post-cardiac arrest patient with poor prognostic features. *Resuscitation*, 2013; 84(6): e81–2.

38. T. Cronberg, M. Brizzi, L.J. Liedholm, et al. Neurological prognostication after cardiac arrest–Recommendations from the Swedish Resuscitation Council. *Resuscitation*, 2013; 84(7): 867–72.

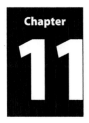

Decompressive Craniectomy for Stroke Patients

Matthew N. Jaffa and David Y. Hwang

Case

Mr. Johnson is a 62-year-old man with no prior past medical history who is admitted to the intensive care unit (ICU) after suffering a large cryptogenic stroke in the past 24 hours, with the majority of his left middle cerebral artery (MCA) now infarcted on neuroimaging. Despite his being globally aphasic with a right hemiparesis, a gaze deviation to the left, and a right-sided hemianopsia, his eyes initially open to voice easily, he has symmetric pupils, and he is protecting his airway. Several hours later in the ICU, the nurse notes that he still has symmetric pupils, but his eyes now require noxious stimulation to open, and he seems to be snoring. His serum sodium is 145 mEq/L; a repeat computed tomography scan of the head (Figure 11.1) shows that he has developed an

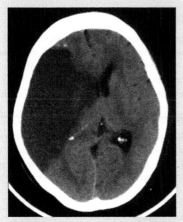

Figure 11.1 Malignant left MCA infarction on a computed tomography scan.

interval increase in cerebral edema and now has a few millimeters of left-to-right midline shift. His family "doesn't want him to die" and is very hopeful that he might improve in the future, saying that he is a very active 62-year-old. You walk into a meeting with the family after ordering mannitol and being told by the nurse that someone on the team had already mentioned the possibility of decompressive craniectomy to them.

Patients with occlusions of the MCA or internal carotid artery and large hemispheric strokes are typically admitted to the ICU for neurologic monitoring. The phrase "malignant MCA syndrome" was first coined in 1996 by Hacke to describe a syndrome of severe hemiparesis and sensory loss, horizontal gaze deviation, and global aphasia (for a dominant hemisphere stroke) that progresses to declining mental and possibly respiratory status over a few days owing to cerebral edema.[1-4] High rates of mortality (approaching 80%) without decompressive craniectomy, as precipitated by compression of the brainstem often occurring within 2 to 5 days of the infarction, are well-documented.[1,2,5] However, determining with neurosurgical colleagues to offer a decompressive craniectomy for an ICU patient with a large hemispheric stroke is often a challenging shared decision for the patient's family, because of the concern of prolonging what may turn out to be a poor quality of life (QoL) for the patient. In this Chapter, we discuss previously completed trials of decompressive craniectomy and consider factors that may inform shared decision-making in these crucial moments.

11.1 Decompression and Outcomes

Several studies and multiple meta-analyses have been completed to understand the role of decompressive craniectomy in the treatment of malignant MCA stroke. These studies all use the modified Rankin Scale (mRS) as a means of quantifying long-term disability, as described in Table 11.1. This ordinal scale starts at 0, indicating no symptoms, and runs to 6, indicating death, with the difference between scores of 3 and 4 being the ability to ambulate and attend to one's own bodily needs without assistance.[6] Scores of 3 and 4 in particular present a challenge when applied to real-life shared decision-making due to the wide array of disability they convey and degree to which this affects a patient's sense of QoL. This challenge has led to an active debate and discussion of how best to judge the impact of intervention in malignant strokes.

11.2 Patients Age 18–60 Years Old

In 2006, enrollment in the Decompressive Craniectomy in Malignant Middle Cerebral Artery Infarcts (DECIMAL)[7] and Decompressive Surgery for the

Table 11.1. Modified Ranking Scale scoring description

The mRS	
0	No symptoms
1	No significant disability, despite symptoms; able to perform usual duties and activities
2	Slight disability; unable to perform all previous activities, but able to look after own affairs without assistance
3	Moderate disability; requires some help, but able to walk without assistance
4	Moderately severe disability; unable to walk without assistance and unable to attend to own bodily needs without assistance
5	Severe disability; bedridden, incontinent, and requires constant nursing care and attention
6	Death

Reprinted from Stroke, vol. 19(5), van Swieten JC, et al. Interobserver agreement for the assessment of handicap in stroke patients, 1988, with permission from Wolters Kluwer Health[6]

Treatment of Malignant Infarction of the Middle Cerebral Artery (DESTINY)[8] studies were aborted prematurely to combine data along with that from Hemicraniectomy After Middle Cerebral Artery infarction with Life-threatening Edema Trial (HAMLET)[9,10] as a meta-analysis, which is now the commonly used dataset cited when discussing outcomes for decompressive craniectomy.[11] Owing to differences in the original eligibility requirements for each study, this meta-analysis included only those subjects between the ages of 18 and 60 with neuroimaging demonstrating infarction in at least 50% of the MCA territory or a volume of greater than 145 mL. Together, 93 patients who had been randomized within 45 hours of symptom onset and intervention completed within 48 hours were included in the meta-analysis.[11]

The primary outcome in the analysis was mRS measured at 12 months and dichotomized to favorable outcome (mRS of 0–4) versus unfavorable (mRS of 5–6), with the recognition that the goal of surgery should be to decrease mortality without an increase in severely disabled survivors. Pooled data demonstrated that decompressive craniectomy decreased rates of death from 71% to 22% and was associated with an absolute risk reduction of 51.2% at 1 year (Figure 11.2).[11] As a secondary aim, results were also dichotomized with favorable outcome being defined as a mRS of 0 to 3 and revealed a significant difference between those in the treatment versus conservative arm, with an absolute risk reduction of 22.7%. Survival with an mRS of 0–3 nearly doubled at 12 months for those in the surgical arm, although ultimately survival with a mRS of 4 increased by nearly 10 times. Before the results of this pooled analysis, there was concern that,

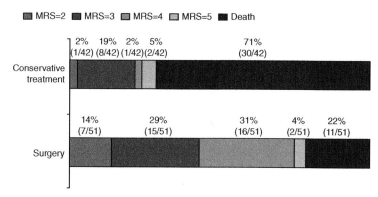

■ MRS=2   ■ MRS=3   ■ MRS=4   □ MRS=5   ■ Death

Figure 11.2 Pooled analysis of the DECIMAL, DESTINY, and HAMLET (1-year patient outcomes) studies.
Reprinted from Lancet, vol. 6(3), Vahedi K, et al. Early decompressive surgery in malignant infarction of the middle cerebral artery: A pooled analysis of three randomized controlled trials, 215–22, 2007, with permission from Elsevier[11]

although decompressive craniectomy could improve rates of survival, the majority of these survivors were left with an mRS of 5. This was not seen in these data, because the rate of survival with an mRS of 5 was equivocal between the study groups.

11.3 Patients Older Than Age 60

Discussion of an age limit for surgical intervention in malignant infarctions is controversial, but frequently discussed among neurologists, neurosurgeons, and intensivists.[12] Although the original trials of decompression focused on younger patients, the DESTINY-2 study was conducted from 2009 to 2013 to assess outcomes in patients older than 60 undergoing decompressive craniectomy.[13]

Enrollment was stopped after 82 patients had reached the 6-month primary outcome, defined as favorable with an mRS of 0–4 versus unfavorable with an mRS of 5 or 6. The results of the primary outcome favored the surgical intervention group with an odds ratio of 2.91 (95% confidence interval, 1.06–7.49; $p = .04$), although of note only 7% of patients in the intervention arm survived with a mRS of 3 or less versus 3% in the conservative arm (Figure 11.3).[13] Survival with severe disability was found in 28% of the intervention group versus only 13% of the conservative treatment arm, although death was documented much less frequently, namely, 33% compared with 70%.

More recently, Streib and colleagues assessed the absolute risk increase in treatment with early craniectomy, allowing them to then calculate the number needed to treat for a defined category of functional outcome and age (Table 11.2).[14]

Table 11.2. Likelihood of different outcomes based on a meta-analysis of six trials

	All Patients		Patients >60 years	
	ARI (%)	NNT	ARI (%)	NNT
Excellent Functional Outcome (mRS 0–2)	6.6	15.2	*	N/A
Favorable Outcome (mRS 0–3)	15.0	6.7	4.0	25.0
Unfavorable Functional Outcome (mRS 4–5)	29.5	3.4	32.5	3.1

ARI = Absolute risk increase; NNT = Number needed to treat. *No patients >60 with mRS 0–2.
Reprinted from Decompressive craniectomy, JM Simard and B Aarabi (eds), MN Jaffa, et al.,
Decompressive Craniectomy for Ischemic Stroke, 197–216, 2018, with permission from Nova Science
Publishers.

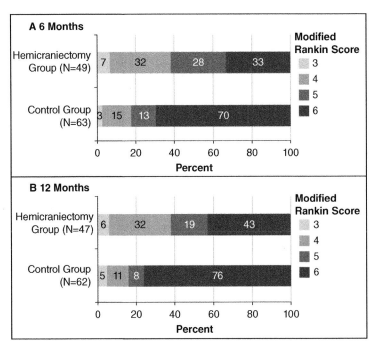

Figure 11.3 Functional outcome after decompressive craniectomy in patients age >60.
From New England Journal of Medicine, Juttler E, et al., Hemicraniectomy in older patients with
extensive middle cerebral artery stroke, Volume 370(12), 1091–100. Copyright © 2014 Massachusetts
Medical Society. Reprinted with permission from Massachusetts Medical Society[13]

11.4 QoL

Each of the previously discussed analyses demonstrate that neurosurgical intervention has an obvious survival benefit in nearly all cases of malignant MCA infarctions; however, the significance of the difference in morbidity between study groups relies on the authors' definition of a "good" outcome. The data can be very helpful to assist in determining the direction of clinical care that we provide, but must be weighed cautiously in relation to the patient's individual beliefs and goals for care.

Trial data do exist that argue that, ultimately, many surviving patients and family members do not regret the decision to undergo surgical intervention, despite their level of disability at the time of follow-up. Among patients in both arms of the DECIMAL trial, 12 of the survivors acknowledged that "life is worth living" all, most, or some of the time; although seven survivors did not complete the QoL measures owing to aphasia and, in one case, refusal.[7] In the DESTINY-2 study, although the rates of depressive symptoms among survivors in both study arms were high, 63% of survivors or caregivers in the surgical arm indicated that they would provide retrospective consent to therapy if given the choice when asked during follow-up visits.[13] A systematic review of trials, cohort, case-control, and case studies of patients with malignant MCA infarctions undergoing decompressive craniectomy demonstrated that QoL scores for survivors averaged 60%–67% on various QoL questionnaires and visual analogue scales.[15]

11.5 Incorporating Outcome Data Into Conversations with Families

Unlike some other disease processes, patients presenting with massive ischemic strokes are very rarely prepared for the sudden disability with which they are left. Seldom have they discussed their wishes with loved ones or documented them in an advance directive, which rarely elaborate beyond the concerns related to terminal illness or vegetative states. For those who have indicated their overarching desires, the circumstances surrounding malignant stroke are unique in a way that family or selected representatives must extrapolate from prior constructs to the specifics of the current medical scenario making the question of how to proceed when intervention may be necessary exceedingly complex. Complicating matters further, the physicians caring for these patients must discuss with the family and patient, if possible, the many varied outcomes that could occur in the setting of potential malignant infarctions early in their disease course.

These conversations are difficult for many reasons, but particularly so because of the complexities in achieving an idealized, substituted judgment

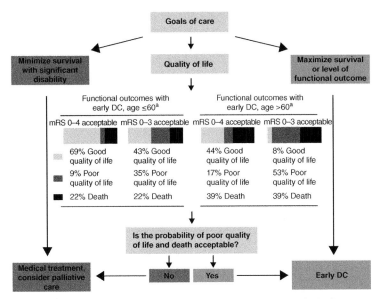

Figure 11.4 Algorithm for hemicraniectomy decision in malignant cerebral infarction as developed by Streib et al.

Reprinted from Neurology Clinical Practice, Vol 6(5), Streib CD, et al., Early decompressive craniectomy for malignant cerebral infarction, 2016 with permission from Wolters Kluwer Health[14]

decision-making framework during a compressed and emotional time. Caution must be practiced to avoid inappropriate framing biases when discussing outcomes while carefully guiding the surrogate decision maker to the best decision for each patient.[16]

The work by Streib and colleagues provides a framework, which can help direct these difficult conversations and questions (Figure 11.4). In their algorithm, patients ages 60 or younger who would consider an mRS of 3 an acceptable QoL have a 43% chance of surviving with such an outcome, a 35% chance of surviving with a poor QoL, and a 22% risk of death. Those who deem an mRS of 4 to be acceptable have a 69% likelihood of good outcome, a 9% chance of poor outcome, and a 22% risk of death.[14] We believe it is important to note that no participant in the trials achieved a mRS of 0 or 1.

11.6 Conclusions

"Malignant" ischemic strokes are associated with an exceptionally high morbidity and mortality. The data would suggest that surgery is an individually applied treatment with the greatest impact on younger patients intervened upon within the first 48 hours of the symptoms.[11,13,14,17-19]

The role of urgent discussion with the family or legally authorized representative for stroke patients at increased risk for the development of malignant edema is paramount. To determine an appropriate direction for care, one ideally needs a firm understanding of what a patient him or herself would have considered to be a satisfactory outcome. Using the clinical decision tree described by Streib provides one method by which care providers can describe the most objective outcome probabilities with the data that is currently available. Collaboration and consistency between neurologists, neurosurgeons, intensivists, and patients' families is critical for establishing treatment plans and goals of care consistent with patients' own wishes.

References

1. W. Hacke, M. Horn, M. Spranger, et al. Malignant middle cerebral artery territory infarction: clinical course and prognostic signs. *Archives of Neurology*, 1996; 53(4): 309–15.

2. J. Hofmeijer, L.J. Kappelle, H.B. van der Worp. Predictors of life-threatening brain edema in middle cerebral artery infarction. *Cerebrovascular Disease*, 2008; 25(1–2): 176–84.

3. B. Hagen, S.S. Huttner. Malignant middle cerebral artery infarction: clinical characteristics, treatment strategies, and future perspectives. *Lancet Neurology*, 2009; 8(10): 949–58.

4. D. Sean Treadwell. Malignant middle cerebral artery (MCA) infarction: pathophysiology, diagnosis and management. *Postgrad Medical Journal*, 2010; 86(1014): 235–42.

5. J.S. Berrouschot, S. Bettin, J. Köster, D. Schneider. Mortality of space-occupying ('malignant') middle cerebral artery infarction under conservative intensive care. *Intensive Care Medicine*, 1998; 24(6): 620–3.

6. J.L. Banks, C.A. Marotta. Outcomes validity and reliability of the modified Rankin scale: implications for stroke clinical trials. *Stroke*, 2007; 38(3): 1091.

7. K. Vahedi, E. Vicaut, J. Mateo, et al. Sequential-design, multicenter, randomized, controlled trial of early Decompressive Craniectomy in Malignant Middle Cerebral Artery Infarction (DECIMAL Trial). *Stroke*, 2007; 38(9): 2506–17.

8. E. Juttler, S. Schwab, P. Schmiedek, et al. Decompressive Surgery for the Treatment of Malignant Infarction of the Middle Cerebral Artery (DESTINY): a randomized, controlled trial. *Stroke*, 2007; 38(9): 2518–25.

9. G.J.A. Hofmeijer, A. Algra, J. van Gijn, et al. Hemicraniectomy after middle cerebral artery infarction with life-threatening Edema trial (HAMLET). Protocol for a randomised controlled trial of decompressive surgery in space-occupying hemispheric infarction. *Trials*, 2006; 7: 29.

10. J. Hofmeijer, L.J. Kappelle, A. Algra, et al, for the HAMLET investigators. Surgical decompression for space-occupying cerebral infarction (the Hemicraniectomy After Middle Cerebral Artery infarction with Life-threatening Edema Trial [HAMLET]): a multicentre, open, randomised trial. *Lancet Neurology*, 2009; 8(4): 326–33.

11. K. Vahedi, E. Juettler, E. Vicaut, et. Early decompressive surgery in malignant infarction of the middle cerebral artery: a pooled analysis of three randomised controlled trials. *Lancet Neurology*, 2007; 6(3): 215–22.

12. E. Juttler, J. Bosel, H. Amiri, et al. DESTINY II: DEcompressive Surgery for the Treatment of malignant INfarction of the middle cerebral arterY II. *International Journal of Stroke*, 2011; 6(1): 79–86.

13. E. Jüttler, A. Unterberg, J. Woitzik, et al., for the DESTINY II Investigators. Hemicraniectomy in older patients with extensive middle-cerebral-artery stroke. *New England Journal of Medicine*, 2014; 370(12): 1091–100.

14. C.D. Streib, L.M. Hartman, B.J. Molyneaux. Early decompressive craniectomy for malignant cerebral infarction meta-analysis and clinical decision algorithm. *Neurology: Clinical Practice*, 2016; 6(5): 433–43.

15. T. van Middelaar, H.B. van der Worp, J. Stam, et al. Quality of life after surgical decompression for space-occupying middle cerebral artery infarction: systematic review. *International Journal of Stroke*, 2015; 10(2): 170–6.

16. T.G. Lukovits, J.L. Bernat. Ethical approach to surrogate consent for hemicraniectomy in older patients with extensive middle cerebral artery stroke. *Stroke*, 2014; 45(9): 2833–5.

17. H.H. Dasenbrock, F.C. Robertson, H. Vaitkevicius, et al. Timing of decompressive hemicraniectomy for stroke: a Nationwide Inpatient Sample analysis. *Stroke*, 2017; 48(3): 704–11.

18. L. Back, A. Kapur, G.D. Eslick. Role of decompressive hemicraniectomy in extensive middle cerebral artery strokes: a meta-analysis of randomised trials. *Internal Medicine Journal*, 2015; 45: 711–17.

19. M.H. Ming-Hao, J. Fu, G. Roodrajeetsing, et al. Decompressive hemicraniectomy in patients with malignant middle cerebral artery infarction: a systematic review and meta-analysis. *Surgeon*, 2015; 13(4): 230–40.

Chapter 12

Decompressive Craniectomy for Traumatic Brain Injury Patients

Connie Ge, Angelos Kolias,
and Susanne Muehlschlegel

Case

Mrs. Smith, a 24-year-old woman without prior past medical history, is admitted to the intensive care unit after a motor vehicle collision with ejection from the vehicle, during which she suffered a severe traumatic brain injury (TBI). The patient was intubated at the scene and remained intubated throughout the hospital course. The patient's Glasgow Coma Scale after resuscitation was 6T (M4, E1, V1(T)). Serial computed tomography (CT) scans of the head revealed left frontal and temporal contusions in evolution with an increasing amount of pericontusional edema, and mass effect with midline shift of the septum pellucidum and compression of the mesencephalic cisterns (Figure 12.1). The patient was treated according to Brain Trauma Foundation guidelines with intracranial pressure (ICP) monitoring for elevated ICP. Initially the patient responded well to medical management with deep sedation, osmotherapy (mannitol and 23.4% hypertonic saline alternating resulting in a serum sodium level of 165 mmol/dL), and normothermia. Sedation holidays were omitted owing to ICPs spiking to 40 mmHg off sedation. On hospital day 5, the patient's ICP continued to intermittently spike to 30 mmHg, and she no longer responded to osmotherapy. A repeat head CT scan revealed an interval increase in the midline shift and pericontusional cerebral edema. Given her age and active lifestyle before the injury, the family wanted "everything done." You call the neurosurgeon and in collaboration with the neurosurgical team you walk into a meeting with the family to discuss secondary decompressive craniectomy (DC) vs. additional medical management with significant potential side effects (induced hypothermia, pentobarbital coma).

TBI remains a major public health issue, as 69 million individuals worldwide suffer a TBI each year[1] and TBI contributes to one third of all injury-related deaths in the United States. Nearly 300,000 TBI-related hospitalizations occur annually in the United States, with more than 56,000 Americans dying annually after sustaining a TBI, of which the majority are due to severe TBI (Glasgow

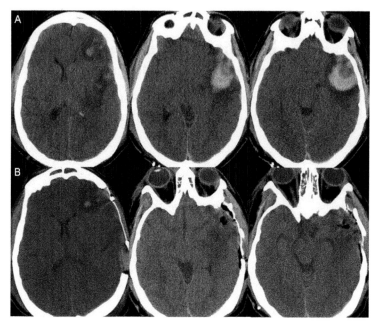

Figure 12.1 Pre- and postcraniectomy head CT scan.
(A) Three slices of the precraniectomy head CT scan of the patient. The patient suffered frontal and temporal hemorrhagic contusions on the left (hyperdense lesions), with pericontusional edema (dark borders), resulting in a left-to-right midline shift of the septum pellucidum, partial compression of the left lateral ventricle, and obliteration of the basal cisterns.
(B) The same three slices of the immediate after craniectomy head CT scan of the same patient, status post left frontotemporal craniectomy and evacuation of the prior left temporal hemorrhagic contusion. The previous midline shift and the compression of the lateral ventricle are improved. The basal cisterns are open.

Coma Scale of ≤8).[2] Additionally, the total number of TBI-related emergency department visits, hospitalizations, and deaths, has increased by 53% since 2006.[3]

Although treatment protocols and management algorithms have been developed over the last two decades for the clinical management of patients with severe TBI,[4–6] the prognostication of outcomes after TBI often remains uncertain. In addition to the limited availability of validated and well-calibrated prediction models,[7,8] physicians have variable confidence in their own accuracy of outcome prediction in TBI[9] and generally low confidence in using the most validated prediction models in patients.[10] Reasons for difficulty with prognostication include that TBI has multiple different pathomechanisms, may co-occur with

Table 12.1. Glasgow Outcome Scale – Extended[12]

1	Death
2	Vegetative state
3	Lower severe disability
4	Upper severe disability
5	Lower moderate disability
6	Upper moderate disability
7	Lower good recovery
8	Upper good recovery

other injuries and complications, and may present implementation and compliance challenges with respect to existing guidelines.[11] In this Chapter, we focus on the use of DC to relieve refractory intracranial hypertension after severe TBI.

12.1 Common Scales Used in TBI

The severity of TBI is graded using the Glasgow Coma Scale, which describes a patient's level of consciousness based on their verbal, motor, and eye-opening responses to stimulus.[12] The most widely used outcome measure has been the 5-point Glasgow Outcome Scale,[13] although more recently, the 8-point extended Glasgow Outcome Scale – Extended (GOS-E) has been shown to have increased sensitivity to small changes in functional status[14] and good reliability, even when administered over the phone.[15] By definition, the GOS-E is an ordinal scale with eight different categories (Table 12.1). The GOS-E is frequently dichotomized into "unfavorable" (GOS-E 1–4) and "favorable" (GOS-E 5–8) outcomes for ease of interpretation in the statistical analysis.[14,16]

12.2 Decompressive Craniectomy

DC refers to the removal of a portion of skull and the opening of the underlying dura to create room for the swollen brain to expand beyond the confines of the cranial vault, thereby relieving intracranial hypertension. DC techniques can be classified in three ways – a unilateral DC (hemicraniectomy) where a large frontotemporoparietal bone flap is removed, a bilateral hemicraniectomy, and a bifrontal DC where the removed bone flap extends from the floor of the anterior cranial fossa to the coronal suture and to the middle cranial fossa floor bilaterally.[17]

"Primary DC" is the use of DC after the evacuation of a space-occupying lesion without replacing the bone flap owing to intraoperative brain swelling or an anticipation that brain swelling will worsen post-operatively, i.e., owing to evolving contusions. "Secondary DC" is used as a part of the tiered management for refractory intracranial hypertension. This event is critical when the patient develops a mass effect from traumatic lesions, resulting in eventual brain herniation and death. Guidelines suggest that, if there is a high index of suspicion that ICP will be elevated in patients who cannot be evaluated clinically, ICP monitoring should be instituted with the goal of maintaining an ICP of less than 23 mmHg and a cerebral perfusion pressure of 60–70 mmHg.[5] Elevated ICP is associated with increased mortality and worse functional status, as well as poor neuropsychological functional outcomes.[18] Medically uncontrollable intracranial hypertension can be managed using DC, mild hypothermia, or barbiturate coma.[4]

12.3 The Role of Secondary DC in TBI

A number of studies in the 1980s and 1990s established the groundwork on the use of DC. These studies showed that patients with a lower ICP had better outcomes,[19] and that DC could be used efficaciously as second-tier therapy.[20]

Jiang et al. published the first multicenter randomized controlled trial in adults assessing the management of refractory intracranial hypertension in 486 patients.[21] This trial suggested that the standard large frontotemporoparietal DC resulted in significantly better ICP control than the smaller diameter temporoparietal DC and was associated with fewer complications and better outcomes. This conclusion has been supported by findings from other studies,[22] and large DC has consequently been recommended.[23]

Most recently, two large, multicenter, randomized controlled trials examined two different hypotheses about the role of DC in refractory intracranial hypertension in severe TBI: (1) the Decompressive Craniectomy in Diffuse Traumatic Brain Injury (DECRA) Trial examined the role of early/neuroprotective bifrontal DC[24] and (2) the Randomized Evaluation of Surgery with Craniectomy for Uncontrollable Elevation of Intracranial Pressure (RESCUEicp) examined the role of unilateral or bifrontal DC as a last-tier therapy for severe and refractory intracranial hypertension.[25]

The DECRA trial randomized 155 patients to receive either bilateral DC or standard of care. All patients received first tier interventions for intracranial hypertension whenever ICP increased to more than 20 mmHg. If the ICP spontaneously increased for more than 15 minutes within 1 hour despite first-tier interventions, patients randomized to surgery underwent large bifrontotemporoparietal DC with bilateral dural opening plus standard care.

Importantly, the DECRA investigators defined "unfavorable outcome" as a GOS-E of 4 or less at 6 months after TBI. In DECRA, patients in the DC group had significantly lower mean ICP, shorter duration of mechanical ventilation, and shorter intensive care unit stays at 6 months, but had higher rates of "unfavorable outcomes" compared with the standard of care control group (70% vs 51%; $p = .02$). This result was likely due to the fact that more patients in the surgery group had bilateral unreactive pupils than the control group (27% vs. 12%; $p = .04$); after post hoc adjustment for baseline pupil reactivity, unfavorable outcome rates were no longer significantly different between the groups.

The RESCUEicp trial took a different approach to examining the role of DC in the management of increased ICP. Investigators assessed DC as a last-tier intervention, enrolling 389 patients who presented with increased ICP of more than 25 mmHg for 1–12 hours despite tier 1 and 2 measures. Patients were randomized to receive either medical management with the option of barbiturates after randomization, or a DC, with the decision about the exact type (i.e., unilateral or bifrontal) dependent on the patients' injury and surgeon discretion. In contrast with DECRA, the predefined primary analysis of RESCUEicp was an ordinal analysis, which is in keeping with recent recommendations.[26] The primary analysis showed a significant between-group difference in the GOS-E distribution and a substantial reduction in mortality with surgery. The prespecified sensitivity analysis dichotomized at upper severe disability (GOS-E ≥ 4) or better was significant at 12 months (i.e., 45% of the patients in the surgical group were at least independent at home, as compared with 32% of patients in the medical group; $p = .01$). At 6 months, the difference in the favorable outcome rates was not statistically significant (43% vs. 35%; $p = .12$).

A comparison of the two studies is informative. The DECRA trial, as compared with the RESCUEicp trial, enrolled patients with a lower ICP threshold (20 mmHg vs. 25 mmHg) for shorter intervals (15 minutes vs. 1–12 hours), and after lower intensities of therapy (stage 1 interventions vs. stage 1 and 2 interventions). At enrollment, the populations also differed with respect to expected outcome, as it has been shown that the requirement for stage 2 interventions increases the relative risk of death by 60%.[27] This fact also accounts for why the pooled mortality of 38% in the RESCUEicp trial vs. 19% in the DECRA trial is unsurprising.

With these conclusions on and new questions raised about the clinical application of DC from these two most recent randomized trials, the International Consensus Meeting on the Role of Decompressive Craniectomy in the Management of Traumatic Brain Injury was organized. Participating delegates met to discuss key topics around DC and published the first consensus statement on the topic.[28] Consensus statements concerning secondary DC are summarized in Table 12.2 .

Table 12.2. Summary of recommendations from the International Consensus Meeting on Secondary Decompressive Craniectomy[28]

(1) ICP monitoring is a necessary part of decision-making for secondary DC.

(2) Secondary DC is effective in decreasing ICP, but underlying brain pathology and pathophysiology contribute to overall outcome.

(3) Secondary DC should be applied selectively owing to uncertainty as to which severe TBI subgroups will truly benefit.

(4) DC may decrease mortality. However, it is not benign and is associated with significant risks of complications and potentially increased risks of disability.

(5) Large DC with opening of the dura is recommended to effectively reduce ICP.

(6) Bifrontal or unilateral DC are options in the surgical treatment of diffuse TBI.

(7) Providers should conduct frank discussions with family members/surrogates regarding the risks, benefits, alternatives, and potential prognosis.

12.4 What Is the Role of Shared Decision-Making in Decompressive Craniectomy?

Patients have the right to make decisions about their own health-care, including whether the risks and benefits of treatment align with their own values and preferences. In the event of severe TBI, patients lack the capacity to make or communicate this decision to physicians, and therefore surrogate decision makers must step in and decide on their behalf.

It is important to consider that in the case of secondary DC, available options are sparse. They include (1) moving forward with DC, (2) not moving forward with DC but continuing aggressive medical management, including pentobarbital coma and hypothermia at some centers, both with substantial potential risks,[25,29] or (3) comfort measures with withdrawal of life-sustaining treatments, which will ultimately result in death.[29] Withdrawal of life-sustaining treatments has been shown to be the greatest predictor of in-hospital mortality for TBI patients,[30] and one multicenter cohort study found that the highly variable rates of mortality after withdrawal of life-sustaining treatments were affected by center rather than by baseline patient characteristics.[31] General critical care research has found physician variability in the decision to limit life support owing to various factors across the categories of physician work environment, physician experiences, physician attitudes, and physician relationships with patients and their families.[32] Additionally, it is critically important that physicians engage in high-quality shared decision-making (SDM) with surrogates because there may exist a self-fulfilling prophecy when considering withdrawal of life-sustaining treatments. Izzy et al. demonstrated in a simulated setting that physicians prognosticate overly pessimistically based on the data available for certain patients, and true hospital discharge and functional outcomes were underestimated by most physicians.[30]

Furthermore, the degree of acceptable disability may differ between individual patients. Although RESCUEicp investigators found that DC was associated with greater positive outcome, it is important to note their unconventional dichotomization of including a GOS-E of 4 as "favorable." Nevertheless, the RESCUEicp investigators justified this as follows[33]:

The severity of injury in the RESCUEicp trial underpinned dichotomization in the prespecified sensitivity analysis at upper severe disability (independent at home) or better. Given the high expectation of a poor outcome, the use of a "conventional" dichotomy would be as inappropriate as the use of it in populations with mild TBI (in whom disability-free survival is often attainable). This approach is concordant with recent recommendations. Upper severe disability is a better outcome than a modified Rankin score of 4 (on a scale from 0 [no symptoms] to 6 [death]), the threshold that has driven the use of craniectomy in patients with ischemic stroke.

In correspondence published in the *New England Journal of Medicine*, the DECRA investigators demonstrated that, with conventional dichotomization of the GOS-E, no differences in outcomes are exhibited in the medical and surgical groups of the RESCUEicp trial,[34] highlighting the need for careful consideration of what outcomes the patient may consider acceptable (Figure 12.2).

This relative subjectivity of the GOS-E has also been expressed by patients themselves. In a study using semi-structured interviews with patients surviving at least 3 years after DC with an unfavorable outcome, the majority of patients stated that they would provide retrospective consent for the procedure.[36] This may be explained in part by the patients' willingness to adjust to a level of disability that was previously unacceptable to them.[37] Although the dichotomization of the GOS-E into favorable and unfavorable seems to imply that the goal of secondary DC is to achieve a favorable outcome, this binary understanding of patient outcomes is known to decrease the sensitivity of the scale, and recent work has examined the use of proportional odds or sliding dichotomy approaches to detect smaller treatment effects.[14] In conversations with families, discussing the range of the possible outcomes without the use of value-laden terms, such as favorable, unfavorable, good, or poor, etc., is probably the way forward. For example, it would be useful explaining that vegetative state and lower severe disability mean that the patient would be dependent on others for care, whereas upper severe disability indicates that the patient is independent at home but requires assistance outside (i.e., for shopping or travelling) and patients classified as having moderate disability are usually employed in a paid or a voluntary capacity, but have not returned to their preinjury employment.[38]

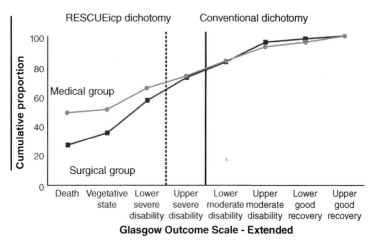

Figure 12.2 Cumulative proportion of patients' GOS-E score.
The cumulative proportion percentage includes all scores lower than the indicated score. Conventional dichotomization (solid line) of the GOS-E defines favorable outcome as moderate disability or good recovery, corresponding with a GOS-E score of 5–8. The RESCUEicp investigators (dotted line) expanded their definition of a favorable outcome to include upper severe disability, corresponding with a GOS-E score of 4–8. Reprinted with permission from Dr. Alistair Nichol.[35]

An emerging number of papers concerning the application of SDM in the critically ill neurologic patient have been published, but a large gap exists between the defined need for SDM and its practical application.[39] Commonly cited barriers include a physician's own limitations with implementing SDM, practical or logistical issues of incorporating SDM, and concerns about passive patients and dominant clinicians.[40] For instance, the increase in a patient's ICP is often an emergent situation and both family and physicians may feel uncomfortable making decisions under the pressing time constraints. There is a high degree of outcome uncertainty and risk associated with DC, and family members of patients who are critically ill may prefer that the physician take a dominant role in decision-making.[41] Although the decision-making process for incapacitated patients differs by country, in the United States families may ultimately choose to withdraw life-sustaining treatment after receiving a secondary DC, with the realization that the patient would not want to live with a tracheostomy and percutaneous feeding tube. This point highlights the importance of discussing the long-term sequelae of DC and not just the immediate surgical risks themselves.[42]

12.5 Conclusions

Secondary DC has been shown to lower mortality after TBI. Because the acceptable level of disability differs between individual patients, clinicians should discuss possible outcomes in an unbiased fashion and include consequences of DC, which often includes tracheostomy/feeding tube placement, and discharge to another long-term acute or subacute care institution. Because in the case of DC and long-term disability after TBI there is no absolute right or wrong answer, SDM is an ideal and preferable approach to be included in the DC consent process. Further research and development of SDM tools will be important to guide both providers and families in caring for patients suffering traumatic brain injury.

References

1. M.C. Dewan, A. Rattani, S. Gupta, et al. Estimating the global incidence of traumatic brain injury. *Journal of Neurosurgery*, 2018; 1: 1–18.

2. A. Christopher, P. Taylor, M Jeneita et al. Traumatic brain injury–related emergency department visits, hospitalizations, and deaths – United States, 2007 and 2013. *MMWR Surveillance Summaries*, 2017; 66.

3. TBI-related Emergency Department Visits, Hospitalizations, and Deaths (EDHDs). 2019. Available: www.cdc.gov/traumaticbraininjury/data/tbi-edhd.html.

4. G.W.J. Hawryluk, S. Aguilera, A. Buki, et al. A management algorithm for patients with intracranial pressure monitoring: the Seattle International Severe Traumatic Brain Injury Consensus Conference (SIBICC). *Intensive Care Medicine*, 2019; 45: 1783–94.

5. N. Carney, A.M. Totten, C. O'Reilly, et al. Guidelines for the management of severe traumatic brain injury, fourth edition. *Neurosurgery*, 2017; 80: 6–15.

6. J. Marehbian, S. Muehlschlegel, B.L. Edlow, et al. Medical management of the severe traumatic brain injury patient. *Neurocritical Care*, 2017; 27: 430–46.

7. E.W. Steyerberg, N. Mushkudiani, P. Perel, et al. Predicting outcome after traumatic brain injury: development and international validation of prognostic scores based on admission characteristics. *PLoS Medicine*, 2008;5:e165; discussion.

8. S.A. Dijkland, K.A. Foks, S. Polinder, et al. Prognosis in moderate and severe traumatic brain injury: a systematic review of contemporary models and validation studies. *Journal of Neurotrauma*, 2020; 37: 1–13.

9. A.F. Turgeon, F. Lauzier, K.E. Burns, et al. Determination of neurologic prognosis and clinical decision making in adult patients with severe traumatic brain injury: a survey of Canadian intensivists, neurosurgeons, and neurologists. *Critical Care Medicine*, 2013; 41: 1086–93.

10. J. Moskowitz, T. Quinn, M.W. Khan, et al. Should we use the IMPACT-Model for the outcome prognostication of TBI patients? A qualitative study assessing physicians' perceptions. *MDM Policy & Practice*, 2018; 3: 2381468318757987.

11. V. Volovici, A. Ercole, G. Citerio, et al. Variation in guideline implementation and adherence regarding severe traumatic brain injury treatment: a CENTER-TBI survey study in Europe. *World Neurosurgery*, 2019; 125: e515–e20.

12. G. Teasdale, B Jennett. Assessment of coma and impaired consciousness. A practical scale. *Lancet*, 1974; 2: 81–4.

13. J.T. Wilson, L.E. Pettigrew, G.M Teasdale. Structured interviews for the Glasgow Outcome Scale and the extended Glasgow Outcome Scale: guidelines for their use. *Journal of Neurotrauma*, 1998; 15: 573–85.

14. J. Weir, E.W. Steyerberg, I. Butcher, et al. Does the extended Glasgow Outcome Scale add value to the conventional Glasgow Outcome Scale? *Journal of Neurotrauma*, 2012; 29: 53–8.

15. A.D. Nichol, A.M. Higgins, B.J. Gabbe, et al. Measuring functional and quality of life outcomes following major head injury: common scales and checklists. *Injury*, 2011; 42: 281–7.

16. D.G. Altman, P Royston. The cost of dichotomising continuous variables. *BMJ*, 2006; 332: 1080.

17. A.G. Kolias, E. Viaroli, A.M. Rubiano, et al. The current status of decompressive craniectomy in traumatic brain injury. *Current Trauma Reports*, 2018; 4: 326–32.

18. S. Badri, J. Chen, J. Barber, et al. Mortality and long-term functional outcome associated with intracranial pressure after traumatic brain injury. *Intensive Care Medicine*, 2012; 38: 1800–9.

19. T. Shishido, K. Nakayama, K. Shojima, et al. A study on the indication of external decompressive hemicraniectomy for acute subdural hematomas. *Neurologia Medico-Chirurigica (Tokyo)*, 1980; 20: 53–60.

20. Z. Rossini, F. Nicolosi, A.G. Kolias, et al. The history of decompressive craniectomy in traumatic brain injury. *Frontiers in Neurology*, 2019; 10: 458.

21. J.Y. Jiang, W. Xu, W.P. Li, et al. Efficacy of standard trauma craniectomy for refractory intracranial hypertension with severe traumatic brain injury: a multicenter, prospective, randomized controlled study. *Journal of Neurotrauma*, 2005; 22: 623–8.

22. W. Qiu, C. Guo, H. Shen, et al. Effects of unilateral decompressive craniectomy on patients with unilateral acute post-traumatic brain swelling after severe traumatic brain injury. *Critical Care*, 2009; 13: R185.

23. X. Huang, L. Wen. Technical considerations in decompressive craniectomy in the treatment of traumatic brain injury. *International Journal of Medical Sciences*, 2010; 7: 385–90.

24. D.J. Cooper, J.V. Rosenfeld, L. Murray, et al. Decompressive craniectomy in diffuse traumatic brain injury. *New England Journal of Medicine*, 2011; 364: 1493–502.

25. P.J. Hutchinson, A.G. Kolias, I.S. Timofeev, et al. Trial of decompressive craniectomy for traumatic intracranial hypertension. *New England Journal of Medicine*, 2016; 375: 1119–30.

26. A.I. Maas, G.D. Murray, B. Roozenbeek, et al. Advancing care for traumatic brain injury: findings from the IMPACT studies and perspectives on future research. *Lancet Neurology*, 2013; 12: 1200–10.

27. N. Stocchetti, C. Zanaboni, A. Colombo, et al. Refractory intracranial hypertension and "second-tier" therapies in traumatic brain injury. *Intensive Care Medicine*, 2008; 34: 461–7.

28. P.J. Hutchinson, A.G. Kolias, T. Tajsic, et al. Consensus statement from the International Consensus Meeting on the Role of Decompressive Craniectomy in the Management of Traumatic Brain Injury: consensus statement. *Acta Neurochirurgerica (Wien)*, 2019; 161: 1261–74.

29. P.J.D. Andrews, H.L. Sinclair, C.G. Battison, et al. European Society of Intensive Care Medicine study of therapeutic hypothermia (32–35°C) for intracranial pressure reduction after traumatic brain injury (the Eurotherm3235Trial). *Trials*, 2011; 12 :8.

30. S. Izzy, R. Compton, R. Carandang, et al. Self-fulfilling prophecies through withdrawal of care: do they exist in traumatic brain injury, too? *Neurocritical Care*, 2013; 19: 347–63.

31. A.F. Turgeon, F. Lauzier, J.F. Simard, et al. Mortality associated with withdrawal of life-sustaining therapy for patients with severe traumatic brain injury: a Canadian multicentre cohort study. *CMAJ*, 2011; 183: 1581–8.

32. M.E. Wilson, L.M. Rhudy, B.A. Ballinger, et al. Factors that contribute to physician variability in decisions to limit life support in the ICU: a qualitative study. *Intensive Care Medicine*, 2013; 39: 1009–18.

33. P.J. Hutchinson, A.G. Kolias, D.K Menon. Craniectomy for traumatic intracranial hypertension. *New England Journal of Medicine*, 2016; 375: 2403–4.

34. D.J. Cooper, A. Nichol, C Hodgson. Craniectomy for traumatic intracranial hypertension. *New England Journal of Medicine*, 2016; 375: 2402.

35. A Nichol. RESCUEicp and the Eye of the Beholder. In: Nickson C, ed. *Life in the Fast Lane.* 2019. Available: https://litfl.com/.

36. S. Honeybul, G.R. Gillett, K.M. Ho, et al. Long-term survival with unfavourable outcome: a qualitative and ethical analysis. *Journal of Medical Ethics*, 2015; 41: 963–9.

37. R.L. Wood, N.A Rutterford. Psychosocial adjustment 17 years after severe brain injury. *Journal of Neurology, Neurosurgery, and Psychiatry*, 2006; 77: 71–3.

38. D.K. Menon, A.G. Kolias, F. Servadei, et al. Survival with disability. Whose life is it, anyway? *British Journal of Anaesthesia*, 2017; 119: 1062–3.

39. S. Muehlschlegel, L. Shutter, N. Col, et al. Decision aids and shared decision-making in neurocritical care: an unmet need in our NeuroICUs. *Neurocritical Care*, 2015; 23: 127–30.

40. H.K. Kanzaria, R.H. Brook, M.A. Probst, et al. Emergency physician perceptions of shared decision-making. *Academic Emergency Medicine*, 2015; 22: 399–405.

41. C. Wilkinson, M. Khanji, P.E. Cotter, et al. Preferences of acutely ill patients for participation in medical decision-making. *Quality & Safety in Health Care*, 2008; 17: 97–100.

42. A.A. Kon, J.E. Davidson, W. Morrison, et al. Shared decision making in ICUs: an American College of Critical Care Medicine and American Thoracic Society Policy Statement. *Critical Care Medicine*, 2016; 44: 188–201.

Chapter 13

Severe Traumatic Spinal Cord Injury

Chris Marcellino and
Alejandro A. Rabinstein

Case

A 43-year-old woman was an unrestrained passenger in a high-speed motor vehicle collision. She was found by emergency medical services to be poorly responsive, with hypotension, mild bradycardia, and hypoventilation, and was intubated at the scene of the accident after a prolonged extrication. A chest tube had been placed based on radiographic findings upon hospital arrival. A computed tomography (CT) scan showed a cervical spine hyperflexion injury with a wedge fracture of the anterior vertebral body of C5 with posterior displacement of the posterior vertebral body and partial compromise of the spinal canal. CT imaging of the head was negative and abdominal and chest imaging showed multiple rib fractures and a subcapsular hematoma of the spleen. Sedation was discontinued shortly after arrival and she was found to have partial activation of the deltoids and elbow flexors, but was otherwise quadriplegic with no motor or sensory function below the C5 level, including absent voluntary anal contraction and perianal sensation. She was triggering the ventilator in a volume control mode. While preparations were made for urgent surgical decompression and stabilization with extensive laminectomy and posterior segmental fusion, magnetic resonance imaging was obtained, which demonstrated extensive cord signal change from C3 to C7 and posterior ligamentous injury, consistent with a flexion-teardrop fracture (Figure 13.1). You are now about to meet the patient's husband to discuss the patient's situation and to obtain consent for the surgery.

13.1 Epidemiology

Traumatic spinal cord injury (SCI) is a major cause of severe neurological disability. It is estimated that there are approximately 200,000 cases of SCI annually worldwide from accidents and violence.[1] In the United States, the annual incidence of SCI is approximately 54 cases per million population or approximately 17,000 new cases each year,[2] with a 4:1 male preponderance.

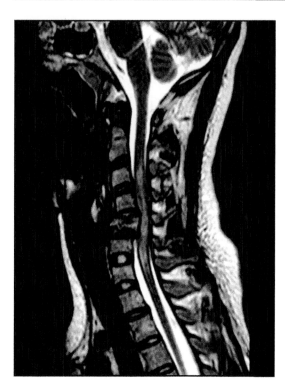

Figure 13.1
Midsagittal T2 magnetic resonance image demonstrating a flexion-teardrop fracture at C5 and spinal cord compression, posterior ligamentous injury and cord signal change from C3 to C6.
(Courtesy Ahmed Abdrabou, MD)

Land vehicle crashes are the leading cause of injury, followed by falls and violence (primarily gunshot wounds). Incomplete tetraplegia is currently the most frequent pattern of injury, followed by incomplete paraplegia, complete paraplegia, and complete tetraplegia. Many individuals with complete high cervical injuries or multiorgan injuries do not survive to receive medical attention and are excluded from these statistics; however, one-half of all SCI involve the cervical spinal cord and produce tetraplegia or tetraparesis.

13.2 Mechanisms of Injury

Traumatic fractures, ligamentous injuries, bony translocation, and direct penetrating injury can result in damage to the spinal cord or conus medullaris. This can range from mild contusions with transient (albeit sometimes profound) neurologic deficits to complete transection of the spinal cord with irrecoverable deficits below the level of injury. Infarction, traumatic disc herniation, stretch injuries, or ligamentous buckling or meningeal rupture can also occur. Blunt or penetrating abdominal trauma with disruption of the blood flow from the aorta or its segmental branches can also produce severe SCI. Myelopathy can extend multiple levels superiorly above the site of compression owing to edema from compression and vascular compromise.

13.3 Neurologic Presentation

Lower motor neuron paralysis at and below the level of the injury is the most common presentation, although the patterns may be incomplete and asymmetric depending on the degree of SCI. Upper motor neuron signs below the level of the injury may develop at a later time.

The American Spinal Injury Association Impairment Scale (AIS or sometimes, ASIA scale) is used to grade and localize SCI with acceptable interrater reliability.[3–5] The severity of injury is denoted by a letter (Table 13.1). An AIS grade of A represents complete loss of motor and sensory function below the level of the lesion, and these cases occur predominantly after high velocity injuries with or without cord transection. However, they can also occur with lower velocity injuries when preexisting spine disease or increased spine rigidity is present, such as with ankylosing spondylitis or after extensive spine fusions.

The initial deficits may be exacerbated by the effects of spinal shock and cord hypoperfusion from neurogenic shock.[6] Neurogenic shock refers to hypotension and poor organ perfusion secondary to interruption of sympathetic autonomic function, resulting in a loss of vasomotor tone, bradycardia owing to unopposed parasympathetic action, and hypothermia. This

Table 13.1. The AIS[5]

Grade	Definition
A	Complete. No sensory or motor function is preserved in the sacral segments S4–S5.
B	Incomplete. Sensory but not motor function is preserved below the neurological level and includes the sacral segments S4–S5.
C	Incomplete. Motor function is preserved below the neurological level, and more then half of key muscles below the neurological level have a muscle grade less then 3 (grades 0–2).
D	Incomplete. Motor function is preserved below the neurological level, and at least half of key muscles below the neurological level have a muscle grade greater than or equal to 3.
E	Normal. Sensory and motor functions are normal.

Used with permission from the American Spinal Injury Association.

hypotension can cause secondary SCI from ischemia and should be promptly reversed. As cord perfusion improves, deficits on examination may improve. In contrast, spinal shock refers to acute stunning of the spinal cord manifested by profound loss of spinal cord function near and distal to the level of injury, including areflexia and autonomic failure.[7,8] Substantial short-term recovery may occasionally occur after resolution of spinal shock, although this occurs more often in younger patients with an initial discrepancy between severe clinical deficits and less severe radiological findings.

13.4 Initial Management of Acute SCI

The initial steps in management include stabilization of the airway, breathing, and circulation, which may be impaired owing to either SCI or associated trauma (i.e., traumatic brain injury, thoracic or abdominal injuries) as well as total spine immobilization with allowance for preservation of any chronic kyphotic deformity. A CT scan of the spine should always be obtained when there is a possible spine injury and the patient has neurological deficits, so as to exclude fractures or gross ligamentous instability warranting surgical evaluation and intervention or bracing. In high energy trauma, an emergent CT scan of the head and torso should also be obtained. Hemodynamic augmentation is recommended to maintain a mean arterial pressure of 85 mmHg or greater for the first 7 days after SCI to minimize secondary injury, though the evidence supporting this recommendation is rather weak.[9–11] The routine use of high-dose methylprednisolone is associated with harmful side effects and is no longer recommended.[12]

Emergency surgery is warranted for mass lesions compressing the spinal cord, such as spinal epidural hematoma or compressive fracture and disc fragments. Otherwise, stabilization of the fractured and unstable spinal column by means of spinal fusion surgery or bracing should be undertaken, ideally within 24 hours of the injury. Until then, the patient should be kept on spinal precautions including strict bedrest, log rolling with turns, and cervical immobilization.

13.5 Discussing Surgical Treatment

When spinal cord compression is ongoing, early surgical decompression is the preferred course of action.[13] The discussion of the need for surgical decompression is often the first decision that gets to be shared with the patient or their surrogates. This discussion inevitably involves considerations of prognosis. Yet, at this early stage, it should be acknowledged that often prognosis cannot be estimated with any certainty.

In the absence of other severe injuries, the patient is often able to provide informed consent and has decision-making capacity. For high cervical injuries and other conditions requiring mechanical ventilation, sedation should be held if feasible to obtain informed consent. When the patient is unable to provide it, consent should be obtained from a surrogate decision maker if one is reachable without undue delay. Otherwise, the physician and surgeon must act in the best interests of the patient guided by the ethical principle of nonmaleficence.

When informing patients or surrogates about the purpose of spine surgery, it should be made clear that decompression may help to improve the deficits, but often the main objective is spine stabilization to prevent further cord injury. When providing consent, patients or their surrogates should not do so expecting postoperative resolution of the deficits. The safety of the surgical intervention based on age, comorbid conditions, and clinical stability should also be reviewed. At the conclusion of the discussion, it should be decided whether the surgery is congruent with the overarching goals of the patient.

Individual factors should be considered when deciding whether to offer surgery. In patients with poor bone quality from osteoporosis or spondyloarthropathy, or any patient with multilevel spinal fractures, longer posterior segmental fusions are often required, which result in longer operative times, greater blood loss, and larger surgical wounds. The cohort of patients who are most likely to require a large surgery (i.e., old and frail patients with extensive comorbidities) are often also those at greatest risk of poor wound healing, surgical site infection, perioperative myocardial infarction, venous thromboembolism, or spinal fusion failure and pseudarthrosis, which can progress to hardware and implant failure, as well as subsequent cord injury. These patients may be considered for palliative bracing after an informed discussion about the risks and benefits of surgery and consideration of the patient's degree of immobility and rehabilitation potential. Alternatively, a more limited surgery or staged surgery may be considered, such as laminectomy for spinal cord decompression alone followed by long-term bracing (i.e., thoracolumbosacral orthosis with or without cervical immobilization or cervical immobilization alone depending on the levels of injury). Long-term bracing is not without risk, because it can lead to skin injuries and ulceration, osteomyelitis, and sepsis. Morbidly obese patients are not good candidates for bracing. Sometimes, the safest treatment is neither surgery nor bracing, and a discussion of the neurological risks and natural history of observation alone is warranted.

13.6 Tracheostomy and Postacute Care of SCI

Patients with high cervical injuries who remain dependent on mechanical ventilation with complete SCI need a tracheostomy for the safe continuation of their care. This represents another critical point in the shared decision-making process. Patients and surrogates should be informed that liberation from mechanical ventilation is very unlikely if no improvement is seen during the acute hospital stay.[14] The appropriateness of tracheostomy and continuation of mechanical ventilation over time in patients who become ventilator dependent depends on how the level of expected long-term disability aligns with the patient's preferences and, to some degree, the patient's optimism regarding future medical and technological advances in SCI. For those patients with decision-making capacity who find (or whose surrogate[s] believe they would find) their degree of disability unacceptable despite education and assistance with adaptation to disability, cessation of mechanical ventilation is an ethically viable option.

During normal swallowing, the larynx is closed and respiration is inhibited. However, this coordination is absent in patients with ventilator dependence. Furthermore, patients with diaphragmatic weakness and impaired cough are unable to clear the respiratory tract and have high rates of aspiration,[15] with subsequent pneumonitis and pneumonia.[16,17] Thus, these patients should undergo gastrostomy tube placement. Gastrostomy may also be needed in milder or lower cervical SCI if assisted feeding is shown to be calorically inadequate or if practical limitations of caretaking make it necessary. Discussing the acceptability of non-oral feeding is thus important when planning for long-term care.

Multidisciplinary rehabilitation with physical and occupational therapy should begin in the ICU as soon as possible.[18] Restrictive pulmonary disease (from neuromuscular weakness), pulmonary and urinary tract infections, venous thromboembolism, fecal impaction, decubitus ulcers and autonomic dysreflexia are also common chronic problems after severe SCI. These expected complications should not only be prevented to the greatest extent possible, but also discussed with patients and surrogates when making decisions about long-term care. Ongoing rehabilitation and some interventions may be quite beneficial in the post-acute stage to improve the quality of life of SCI survivors. For instance, patients with lower cervical spine injuries may benefit from tendon transfer surgery, which often allows these patients to regain better proximal function of the upper extremities.[19]

13.7 Prognosis

Most of the functional recovery after SCI takes place within the first year of injury; however, there is considerable heterogeneity. Mortality is associated with the severity of injury (AIS grade) and age (Table 13.2). Paraplegics can expect a normal life span; while the 10-year mortality of patients who suffer

Table 13.2. Life expectancy in years (after injury) by severity of SCI and age at injury[2]

Age at injury	No SCI	For persons who survive the first 24 hours					For persons who survive the first 1 year				
		AIS D	Para	Low tetra (C5–C8)	High tetra (C1–C4)	Ventilator dependent	AIS D	Para	Low tetra (C5–C8)	High tetra (C1–C4)	Ventilator dependent
20	59.5	52.6	45.1	40.0	35.7	19.3	52.9	45.5	40.7	36.9	25.3
40	40.6	34.2	27.7	23.5	20.1	8.9	34.5	28.1	24.1	21.0	12.6
60	23.1	17.9	13.1	10.3	8.1	2.2	18.2	13.4	10.6	8.7	4.0

Used with permission from the National Spinal Cord Injury Statistical Center (NSCISC.) Publication Disclaimer: The NSCISC provides access to data under a grant from the National Institute on Disability, Independent Living, and Rehabilitation Research (NIDILRR grant number 90DP0083). NIDILRR is a Center within the Administration for Community Living (ACL), Department of Health and Human Services (HHS). The contents of this publication do not necessarily represent the policy of NSCISC, NIDILRR, ACL, and HHS, and you should not assume endorsement by the Federal Government.

SCI with quadriplegia after age 50 approaches 50%. Patients who remain ventilator dependent have approximately one-half the life expectancy of those with otherwise comparable injuries who are not ventilator dependent. Rehospitalizations are frequent and often owing to genitourinary or respiratory infections, venous thromboembolism, or complications from skin ulceration. Yet, and very importantly, patients with tetraplegia generally report satisfaction with the long-term quality of their life.[19,20] It is therefore crucial to emphasize that most individuals acquire coping mechanisms that allow them to enjoy life in different ways than before despite the residual disability.

Many innovative therapies are under investigation for the treatment of patients with sequelae from SCI, including neuroprotective medications, stem cell-based treatments, and electrical neuromodulation. However, none of these interventions can currently be recommended as a part of clinical practice. Patients and families often learn about these investigational treatments and sometimes contact centers where they are being offered commercially. It is, therefore, prudent to educate patients and families about these potentially harmful and even predatory practices.

13.8 Conclusion

Shared decision-making is crucial for informed consent before spine surgery for decompression or stabilization, especially in patients with high surgical risk or who have very poor bone quality, and when contemplating the decision to proceed with tracheostomy and gastrostomy. The level of expected long-term disability must be aligned with the individual patient's preferences when deciding on prolonged life-sustaining artificial measures. However, patients must be made aware of studies showing that even patients with severe and permanent disability from SCI report satisfactory quality of life years after the injury.

References

1. B. Lee, R.A. Cripps, M. Fitzharris, et al. The global map for traumatic spinal cord injury epidemiology: Update 2011, global incidence rate. *Spinal Cord*, 2014; 52(2): 110.

2. *Spinal cord injury (SCI) facts and figures at a glance.* Birmingham, AL: National Spinal Cord Injury Statistical Center; 2016.

3. S. Kirshblum, W. Waring. Updates for the international standards for neurological classification of spinal cord injury. *Physical Medicine and Rehabilitation Clinics*, 2014; 25(3): 505–17.

4. T.T. Roberts, G.R. Leonard, D.J. Cepela. Classifications in brief: American spinal injury association (ASIA) impairment scale. *Clinical Orthopaedics and Related Research*, 2017; 475(5): 1499–504.

5. Association ASI. *Standards for neurological classification of spinal injury patients.* Chicago: American Spinal Injury Association; 1984.

6. P.P. Atkinson, J.L. Atkinson, editors. *Spinal shock.* Mayo Clinic Proceedings. New York: Elsevier, 1996.

7. G. Guillain, J. Barre. Étude anatomo-clinique de quinze cas de section totale de la moelle. *Annals of Medicine*, 1917; 2: 178–222.

8. M. Hall. Synopsis of the diastaltic nervous system. Being the Croonian Lectures, delivered at the Royal College of Surgeons. *Lancet*, 1850; 55(1395): 615–7.

9. F.L. Vale, J. Burns, A.B. Jackson, et al. Combined medical and surgical treatment after acute spinal cord injury: results of a prospective pilot study to assess the merits of aggressive medical resuscitation and blood pressure management. *Journal of Neurosurgery*, 1997; 87(2): 239–46.

10. L. Levi, A. Wolf, H. Belzberg. Hemodynamic parameters in patients with acute cervical cord trauma: description, intervention, and prediction of outcome. *Neurosurgery*, 1993; 33(6): 1007–17.

11. B.C. Walters, M.N. Hadley, R.J. Hurlbert, et al. Guidelines for the management of acute cervical spine and spinal cord injuries: 2013 update. *Neurosurgery*, 2013; 60(Suppl 1): 82–91.

12. M.B. Bracken, M.J. Shepard, W.F. Collins, et al. A randomized, controlled trial of methylprednisolone or naloxone in the treatment of acute spinal-cord injury: results of the Second National Acute Spinal Cord Injury Study. *New England Journal of Medicine*, 1990; 322(20): 1405–11.

13. J.M. Liu, X.H. Long, Y. Zhou, et al. Is urgent decompression superior to delayed surgery for traumatic spinal cord injury? A meta-analysis. *World Neurosurgery*, 2016; 87: 124–31.

14. J.W. McDonald, C. Sadowsky. Spinal-cord injury. *Lancet* 2002; 359(9304): 417–25.

15. C. Wolf, T. Meiners. Dysphagia in patients with acute cervical spinal cord injury. *Spinal Cord*, 2003; 41(6): 347–53.

16. E. Chaw, K. Shem, K. Castillo, et al. Dysphagia and associated respiratory considerations in cervical spinal cord injury. *Topics in Spinal Cord Injury Rehabilitation*, 2012; 18(4): 291–9.

17. R. Abel, S. Ruf, B. Spahn. Cervical spinal cord injury and deglutition disorders. *Dysphagia*, 2004; 19(2): 5–94.

18. A.A. Rabinstein. *Traumatic Spinal Cord Injury. Neurological Emergencies.* New York; Springer; 2020. pp. 271–80.

19. K.S. Wuolle, A.M. Bryden, P.H. Peckham, et al. Satisfaction with upper-extremity surgery in individuals with tetraplegia. *Archives of Physical Medicine and Rehabilitation*, 2003; 84(8): 1145–9.

20. B.W. Chase, T.A. Cornille, R.W. English. Life satisfaction among persons with spinal cord injuries. *Journal of Rehabilitation*, 2000; 66(3): 14.

Potentially Inappropriate Treatment and Conscientious Objection

Nneka O. Sederstrom and
Alexandra Wichmann

The moral ends of medicine established thousands of years ago through the work of historical figures like Imhotep and Hippocrates taught us what it means to be a healer and a clinician. Imhotep embodied being a physician; Hippocrates outlined our duties. Today, we focus on patient-centered care. We strive to provide the best possible care options, even when that means caring while they die. Providing a carefully considered treatment plan that focuses on symptom management, comfort measures, and quality of life is both good medicine and a necessary component of ethically appropriate care. The ability to provide appropriate interventions and transition to comfort care in a timely manner is often difficult. This Chapter explores the issues surrounding requests for potentially inappropriate treatments, the feelings of clinician obligation to respect patient/surrogate autonomy, the inherent conflict between physician autonomy and patient/surrogate autonomy, and how to use a seven-step conflict resolution process to address irreconcilable discord.

Case

A 27-year-old patient with cystic fibrosis arrived in the emergency department with his mother and wife, and complaining of dyspnea and respiratory distress. He was found to be in acute respiratory failure requiring intubation with right-sided pneumothorax necessitating chest tube placement. A subsequent workup found carbapenem-resistant *Pseudomonas aeruginosa* pneumonia, leading to septic shock requiring multiple pressors. The patient was well-known to the pulmonary service as a "noncompliant" clinic patient who frequently missed appointments and skipped tests for potential lung transplant workup. On arrival, the nurses noted that the patient's wife seemed to have "slurred speech, droopy eyes, and an unsteady gait." The patient was stabilized and admitted to the intensive care unit (ICU). During the first 3 days of the hospital stay, his wife was seen sporadically and evaluated by nursing as "incapacitated due to apparent alcohol and drug use." During chart review, they noticed a note from a previous stay discussing an altercation between the wife and the patient's mother for unknown reasons requiring intervention by hospital security.

The critical care attending decided the patient's mother would be the best decision maker, but she refused to agree with the outlined plan of care, instead demanding incorrect interventions. The mother agreed and consented for tracheostomy placement on intubation day 25. The patient's neurologic function did not improve as expected; he opened his eyes and moved only in response to pain. Kidney damage sustained during septic shock worsened, and the patient was diagnosed with end-stage renal disease and was placed on hemodialysis. He was also found to have worsening right-sided heart failure from his chronic pulmonary disease, and the heart failure team was consulted.

After evaluation by the heart failure service, they determined his condition was reversible with time. This team continually validated the possibility for the patient to return to prior baseline despite the new diagnoses of ventilator-dependent respiratory failure and end-stage renal disease. The critical care team felt the prognosis was poor and sought out prognostic opinions from the other care teams, including pulmonary, nephrology, and primary care. All other teams deemed the prognosis to be poor with no anticipated meaningful recovery in functional status, and recommended transitioning goals of care to comfort without escalation of aggressive interventions. Despite multiple interdisciplinary care meetings, the heart failure service continued to recommend aggressive interventions, including referral for a right ventricular assist device. The patient's mother refused to engage in discussions with the primary team or discussions with the palliative care team to initiate comfort measures. She insisted that her son was a "fighter" and the ICU team needed to "do everything." This created an ethical conflict with three components: (1) providing medically appropriate comfort care and hospice to a patient suffering from a nonsurvivable condition, (2) dealing with a surrogate decision maker who has demonstrated repeated intransigence and absolutism in her son's care, and (3) dealing with other clinical colleagues who disagree with the prognosis and continue to offer interventions contradictory to the primary team's plan of nonescalation and withdrawal.

14.1 Determining Appropriate Decision Makers and Patient Autonomy

The case presented highlights a common ethical dilemma around identifying the appropriate decision maker for a patient. Ideally, a patient is fully able to engage in a therapeutic relationship with the clinical team and partner in decision-making. This process of shared decision-making is the best way to respect patient autonomy and should be the standard for all situations where capacity is not of concern.[1] In cases where capacity is called into question, assessing for decision-making capacity is mandated. Most states have laws dictating who is allowed to determine capacity, although any physician can evaluate a patient for capacity to make medical decisions.[2] If a patient lacks capacity, the clinical team should not have conversations about the goals of care or medical interventions with just anyone from the patient's life. Only a life-threatening emergency grants exemption from this principle, allowing providers to provide necessary care immediately. In all other cases, although it can be onerous, there is time to determine who in the patient's life is the most appropriate surrogate decision maker. ICUs should have processes to determine the appropriate decision maker and engage her or him within a reasonable time after admission, the standard being 24–48 hours following admission.[1] In the case presented herein, the ICU physician appropriately decided that the mother was the appropriate surrogate based on the patient's incapacity, the wife's unstable behavior and chemical dependency, and the legal right for the patient's mother to be considered an appropriate surrogate.

14.2 Clinician Autonomy and Clinical Decision-Making

It is oftentimes assumed that the clinical team does not have its own autonomy for decision-making and must comply with all requests from a patient and/or surrogate in order to be compliant in respecting patient autonomy, even if the request requires the clinician to compromise her or his personal values. Clinicians, as autonomous agents themselves, have the right to accept or refuse requests to perform interventions against which they have a moral objection – the sticking point being the maintenance of patient safety and upholding the adage of *primum non nocere*. A physician's ability to opt out of providing objectionable treatments for religious or moral reasons has been reinforced by state and federal laws, as well as by the American Medical Association's Code of Medical Ethics.[3] These opt-out clauses assume a nonemergent situation that allows for alternative physicians to replace the objecting physician. In the reality of urgent ICU situations where no other qualified physician may be available, the ethical duty to treat according to the best interest of the patient takes precedence, and personal objection may be forfeited.

14.3 Conflicting Autonomy: Clinician vs. the Patient/Surrogate

In the case as presented, the primary ICU team evaluated the patient and provided all the additional subspecialty opinions necessary to fully describe what they understand his diagnosis and prognosis to be. During their treatment and evaluation, the patient's mother – as his appropriate surrogate – did not assist in decision-making. She refused interventions deemed necessary, requested medications that were considered inappropriate and potentially dangerous, and repeatedly refused to discuss the goals of care. For the patient's mother, she saw her duty as protecting her son from "bad" interventions. She fought for care that made sense to her and, as she later noted, she wanted to give her "fighter" son every opportunity to heal. Additionally, her beliefs were validated by the heart failure team, which likely increased her confidence as her son's surrogate. The lens through which this situation is viewed is crucial. We tend to focus on the viewpoint that best aligns with our own opinion, without taking the time to better understand any others. Using supporting services like social work, spiritual care, and ethics may help each party to appreciate the values, goals, and wishes of the other. Despite the conflict, both the clinicians and the surrogate want what is best for the patient. Keeping this reality at the forefront gives the best chance of success when working towards common objectives.

Despite all parties having a desire for a "quick fix" to these conflicts, many times there really is not an easy way out. It takes time, energy, emotion, and compromise to resolve such difficult situations. Neither side "wins" when there is contention in the relationship. Clinicians do not always have to grant the patient/surrogate requests, nor does the surrogate/patient always have to accept the therapy presented by the clinicians. Respecting autonomy for both these agents requires time investment to better understand where values are conflicting and where communication is breaking down.

Because time is always a limited resource in the ICU, enlisting the help of supportive services can catalyze this process, but the primary responsibility still rests with the ICU team. Dangerous risks of handing off this duty to others promotes increasing distrust while sabotaging the physician-patient relationship. If conflict continues despite best efforts at resolution, using a seven-step conflict resolution process developed by several of the major scientific and clinical societies is recommended (Figure 14.1).[4]

Starting the conflict resolution process requires ensuring the situation meets certain criteria (Table 14.1).

According to Kon et al. (2016)[5]:

> ICU interventions should generally be considered inappropriate when there is no reasonable expectation that the patient will improve sufficiently to survive outside the acute care setting, or when there is no reasonable expectation that the patient's neurologic function will improve sufficiently to allow the patient to perceive the benefits of treatment.

In this case, regardless of other clinicians' recommendations, if the outcome is not advancing the goal to "survive outside the acute care setting," those recommendations should not be offered. It is also possible that this patient will never recover neurologic function to perceive the benefits of additional aggressive interventions. Therefore, it is acceptable to conclude that aggressive interventions are not medically appropriate and should not be offered or performed.

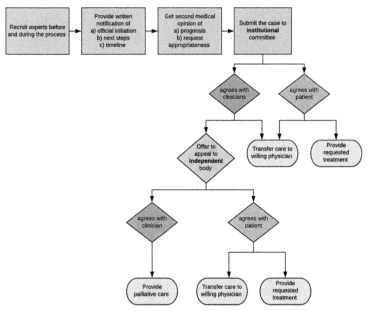

Figure 14.1 Recommended steps for resolution of conflict regarding potentially inappropriate treatments.
Reprinted from Critical Care Medicine, Vol 44(9), Kon AA, et al., Defining futile and potentially inappropriate interventions: A policy statement from the Society of Critical Care Medicine Ethics Committee, 2016 with permission from Wolters Kluwer Health.[5]

14.4 Conclusion: Solving the Case

Working with the patient's mother to find a mutually agreed-upon resolution would be ideal. In most cases, continued conversations from physicians and supportive services help the family adjust to their loved one's end-of-life situation and can decrease conflict. However, when the conflict is entrenched, working through the seven-step process can be of great utility. If the patient starts to decline during the conflict resolution process, it is ethically and medically reasonable to only provide interventions in line with the goals established, such as comfort care with no further escalation, respecting clinician autonomy. The surrogate needs to be informed that the physicians will continue to maintain comfort without adding further invasive interventions. As always, patients and surrogates have the right to transfer to another facility if it is safe and if another physician is willing to accept.

Importantly, clinicians must feel supported by the administration in upholding their clinical duties to provide only care that is beneficial to

Table 14.1. Recommendations from Defining Futile and Potentially Inappropriate Interventions

1. Appropriate goals of ICU care include:
   a. Treatment that provides a reasonable expectation for survival outside the acute care setting with sufficient cognitive ability to perceive the benefits of treatment.
   b. Palliative care that provides comfort to patients through the dying process may be an appropriate goal of care in some ICUs.

2. ICU interventions should generally be considered inappropriate when there is no reasonable expectation that the patient will improve sufficiently to survive outside the acute care setting, or when there is no reasonable expectation that the patient's neurologic function will improve sufficiently to allow the patient to perceive the benefits of treatment.

3. These definitions should not be considered exhaustive. There will be cases in which life-prolonging interventions may reasonably be considered inappropriate even when the above definition is not met.

4. Decisions regarding whether specific interventions are inappropriate should be made on a case-by-case basis.

5. The term "futile" should be used only in the rare circumstance that an intervention simply cannot accomplish the intended physiologic goal. Clinicians should not provide futile interventions and should carefully explain the rationale for the refusal, a process-based approach should be used whenever an intervention is considered potentially inappropriate yet the patient or surrogate decision-maker(s) requests the intervention.

6. A process-based approach should be used whenever an intervention is considered potentially inappropriate yet the patient or surrogate decision-maker(s) requests the intervention.

7. When time pressures make it infeasible to complete all seven steps and the above definition is met, clinicians should refuse to provide the requested treatment and endeavor to complete as much of the seven-step process as the clinical situation allows. Such a decision is consistent with professional standards and good medical practice.

8. At times, it may be appropriate to provide time-limited ICU interventions to a patient even when the above definition is met if doing so furthers the patient's reasonable goals of care.

9. If the patient is experiencing pain or suffering, treatment to relieve pain and suffering is always appropriate.

patients, even when that duty is at odds with an unrealistic perception by the family. Doing what is right includes providing pain and symptom relief, comfort-directed care, and withdrawing burdensome interventions that do not support the goal of achieving a peaceful death. Supporting and cradling families while they grieve is necessary; chaplains and social work professionals serve effectively as members of the care team and should be consulted earlier rather than later to establish rapport and assist where clinicians may falter. Enabling the opportunity for the family to grieve and spend time with the patient is also a key component of the physician's obligation to care for patients and families.

Although the axiom of *primum non nocere* can be complicated in certain clinical scenarios, striving toward this goal will bring clinicians and surrogates to center on that which is best for the patient.[6]

References

1. A.A. Kon, J.E. Davidson, W. Morrison, et al. Shared decision making in ICUs: An American College of Critical Care Medicine and American Thoracic Society policy statement. *Critical Care Medicine*, 2016; 44(1): 188–201.

2. C. Barstow, B. Shahan, M. Roberts. Evaluating medical decision-making capacity in practice. *American Family Physician*, 2018; 98(1): 40–6.

3. American Medical Association. Opinion 1.1.2 Prospective Patients. Code of Medical Ethics. Available: www.ama-assn.org/delivering-care/ethics/prospective-patients. (Accessed December 19, 2019).

4. G.T. Bosslet, T.M. Pope, G.D. Rubenfeld, et al. An official ATS/AACN/ACCP/ESICM/SCCM policy statement: responding to requests for potentially inappropriate treatments in intensive care units. *American Journal of Respiratory and Critical Care Medicine*, 2015; 191(11): 1318–30.

5. A.A. Kon, E.K. Shepard, N.O. Sederstrom, et al. Defining futile and potentially inappropriate interventions. *Critical Care Medicine*, 2016; 44(9): 1769–74.

6. D.K. Sokol. "First do no harm" revisited. *BMJ*, 2013; 347: f6426.

Shared Decision-Making in Emergent Situations

Katharine R. Colton and Evie G. Marcolini

Case

Ms. Patterson is a 68-year-old woman with a history of hypertension who was at home when she developed a sudden-onset severe headache with vomiting. She called 911 but was obtunded on arrival of emergency medical services and could give no further history. She was brought to the emergency department (ED) within 40 minutes of the onset of headache. On arrival to the ED, her blood pressure is 205/110 mmHg and her heart rate is 90; she is taking shallow breaths with a respiratory rate of 32 breaths per minute with an oxygen saturation of 94%. She has a fixed pupil on the left and does not withdraw from painful stimulus on the right. Her family arrives 20 minutes later, and by then a computed tomography (CT) scan has been performed, showing a 7-cm intracerebral hemorrhage (ICH) with a "spot sign" on the CT angiogram. The spot sign describes an area of contrast enhancement within a hemorrhage that serves as an independent predictor of ICH expansion and poor outcome. On return from the CT, she has a Glasgow Coma Scale of 7.

Patients presenting to the ED with acute, severe illness are in a particularly vulnerable position. They, or their surrogates, are asked to make meaningful medical decisions often while in significant pain or distress. Emergency physicians (EPs) are often asked to care for unstable, acutely ill patients with incomplete information and only a short amount of time to establish trust and guide management.

15.1 Capacity

The capacity for decision-making about medical treatment requires that the patient be able to comprehend enough information about the decision at hand, as well as the consequences of each option. The patient should be able to weigh the risks and benefits of each choice compared to her own values and be able to communicate that choice.

Because our patient does not have the capacity to make or communicate her own decision, the EP needs to determine a surrogate to represent her wishes.

15.2 Surrogacy

The patient may have already prepared an advance directive document that establishes who can make medical decisions in their stead and/or what parameters they would want if they could make the decision. But the reality is that most healthy adults have not completed an advance directive or living will.[1]

In the absence of an established medical surrogate, or parameters for goals of care in the situation of end-of-life decision-making, the EP must turn to the state statutes on surrogacy. Each state provides guidance as to who may legally act as a surrogate, or decision maker, unless he or she waives the right to this.[2] Surrogacy law varies from state to state. If there are no family surrogates available, the medical team, usually represented by a social work or case management professional, will petition the state to take legal guardianship.

Surrogates vary widely with respect to their preference to be in complete control of decisions vs. looking to the physician to guide decisions.[3,4] The EP, in only a limited period of time must determine what decisions need to be made, who the surrogate is, what their level of understanding is for medical issues and what their preference for decision-making will be. These preferences may be influenced by religion, ethnicity, culture and/or region.

Of course, these processes all take time, and in the ED in the midst of multiple patients each with critical decisions regarding life support there is rarely that kind of time.

So what to do?

15.3 The Unique ED Environment

The principles of critical decision-making are different in the ED compared with any other aspect of the healthcare environment. Acute phase critical illness in the ED forces time-pressured decisions. A patient's pathophysiology may be associated with uncertain prognosis. Relevant to our case, we know that early prognostication in the case of devastating brain injury can be highly inaccurate and that withdrawal of life sustaining therapies in the first hours may indeed determine mortality.[5–7]

In some cases, the family will accompany the patient and have an abundance of information about the patient, including her medical history, values, wishes, and other nuanced therapeutic limitations such as no consent for blood transfusion. However, in many other cases, the patient may arrive alone, or even unidentified, with no evidence of her background, medical history or goals of care. In most hospitals in the United States, once a patient is identified, demographic and medical information can be found in the electronic medical record. Without background information, critical decisions default to the most conservative, which may not be in concert with the patient's wishes.

One of the unique challenges for the EP is to get to know the patient and/or family in a very short period of time while simultaneously guiding the evaluation, diagnosis, and treatment of the patient. This process differs from the inpatient or outpatient setting, where there is more often ample time during the admission or over a prolonged patient–physician relationship to get to know the patient, their medical issues, values, and goals for care. The EP must quickly establish both knowledge of the patient and trust with the family, as well as determine how to educate the family on the pathophysiology, complications and expectations associated with each disease process.

In a case like the one presented here, with a sudden onset of a devastating injury, and in the setting of no prepared guidance, surrogates often default to considering what values were most important to the patient, or what they think the patient would say if she could communicate in real time with the contemporary knowledge of her injury. This does not take into account the possibility that the patient, or any of us, might look at quality of life decisions differently in the face of a devastating injury than we do when we are in good health.[8] This "disability paradox" attempts to explain the gulf between self-reported acceptable or even excellent quality of life in individuals with disability and the undesirable existence they are perceived to have by others.[9]

Particularly in neurologic emergencies, early prognostication shapes subsequent medical care with the intention of avoiding futile, painful, and costly care in those with an inevitable poor outcome. The author of the original ICH score, developed as a clinical grading tool, but frequently used to communicate prognosis or even triage intervention, has cautioned against the self-fulfilling prophecy of a perceived poor outcome.[10] In the absence of an underlying terminal condition or clearly stated wishes, clinician perception of a potentially poor prognosis should not preclude a reasonable trial of aggressive treatment.

Case, Continued

Ms. Patterson's two eldest daughters arrive and are at the bedside, requesting an update. They are both distressed at their mother's lack of response to questions and sonorous respirations. They do not know whether their mother has an advance directive, but one recalls how difficult it had been for their mother to watch their father suffer through a critical illness several years prior.

15.4 Advance Care Planning

When available, documentation of a patient's choices or priorities before a crisis can inform time-pressured decisions in medically complex or fragile patients. Multiple models for advance care planning exist and can include standing do not resuscitate (DNR) and do not intubate (DNI) orders, durable powers of attorney, and advance directives (see Chapter 16, "Advance Directives: Law, Policy, and Use in Shared Decision-Making). These documents have become more common among elderly patients in the last two decades, although this trend shows negligible association with hospitalization or death in a hospital, suggesting that completing these forms may not significantly change a patient's trajectory.[11] In contrast, the Physician Orders for Life-Sustaining Treatment (POLST) paradigm – also known by a host of similar acronyms including POST, MOLST, MOST, COLST – has been shown to decrease unwanted intervention. POLST forms were developed to address the shortcomings of more cursory advance directives and are associated with decreased rates of in-hospital death and field resuscitation.[12,13] Although an advance directive can identify medical therapies a patient would or would not want, POLST can translate these wishes into medical orders in the ED and help to guide recommendations.

Although a POLST document can help to clarify overarching treatment goals, EPs must take care not to generalize specific directives, including DNR/DNI orders. Multiple studies have shown that patients with a DNR order receive less aggressive care and are significantly more likely to die during admission.[14] In one study of patients admitted with acute myocardial infarction, 44% of those with a DNR died vs. 5% of those without.[15] Further muddying the waters, several studies have found rates of discordance between documented wishes and informed consent to be upwards of 30%–50%.[16,17] These ambiguities leave many EPs in the position of defaulting to full resuscitation. Recently, several cases have caught the media's attention with nonstandard advance directives – in one example, an unconscious patient with a "Do Not Resuscitate" tattoo across his chest.[18] Without further information about the patient's underlying motives, EPs should default to medically appropriate resuscitation.

Case, Continued

Ms. Patterson remains minimally responsive, although her oxygen saturation is appropriate with supplementation via nasal cannula. To her daughters, you bring your concern that she may need endotracheal intubation in the near future. They ask whether this will improve the chances that she returns to a normal life; she had expressed in the past that she would not wish to be kept alive "on life support."

15.5 Shared Decision-Making

In many cases, some decisions are time sensitive, while others may be deferred.[19] In our example, with the patient's Glasgow Coma Scale of 7, we can argue that endotracheal intubation, by general emergency medicine standards, is necessary to protect from aspiration. But in the case of a brain-injured patient, the Glasgow Coma Scale is significantly decreased by virtue of her inability to move right-sided extremities, and it is possible that she retains the ability to protect her airway. We can argue that the benefit of not intubating her (to give the surrogate more time to determine what her wishes would be with more certainty) is outweighed by the benefit of not performing an invasive procedure that she would not have wanted, despite the small risk of aspiration and resulting pneumonia. In contrast, we could argue that withdrawing the endotracheal tube after determination that she would not have wanted it is legally, ethically, and morally the same as not having placed it in the first place. The challenge for the EP is to be able to clearly and succinctly discuss issues such as this with the surrogate in a way that enables him/her to make an appropriate decision for the patient.[3]

A wrenching episode of the podcast "Hidden Brain," aired in November 2019,[20] that told the story of a family left reeling after their wife and mother's diagnosis of amyotrophic lateral sclerosis and subsequent decline. As a nurse, she had cared for many people facing grave illness and death; she had privately told her family many times that she would not accept the quality of life she saw in these encounters. After her diagnosis with a progressive and fatal disease, her family assumed these wishes would remain constant. When faced with the inevitable crisis, her husband was shocked when she assented to an emergent tracheostomy to provide permanent ventilation. Their story is disquieting and illustrates the tension between the priorities we think we hold dear and the will to survive, to get one more day.

15.6 Creating a Structure for Time-Limited Conversations with Family in Emergency Situations

The challenges discussed must be met in the setting of an ED that may be very busy, and with or without the assistance of ancillary staff such as a surgical specialist, social work, case management or clergy. The EP should structure conversations with a family or surrogate to prioritize communication of the diagnosis, identify immediate decisions to be made, and implement a shared plan. A recent qualitative study of ED patients/surrogates and their perception of shared decision-making concluded that a primary barrier to the process was a lack of patient awareness that they could be involved in medical decisions.[21] We recommend making this process explicit with an invitation to participate, free of medical jargon.

Communication of the patient's medical condition is crucial, because conveying the medical findings and diagnosis lays the foundation for the rest of the conversation. Patient decision aids, when available, are known to increase patient comprehension[22] and may prove particularly helpful for patients or surrogates with low health literacy.[23] A well-designed visual aid uses clear language and graphics that help to contextualize relatively complex decisions. An excellent example is put forward by Ouchi et al.,[24] in which they create a simple graphic to show eventual outcomes in elderly patients undergoing intubation in the ED (Figure 15.1).

Older adults can expect the following after an emergency department intubation:

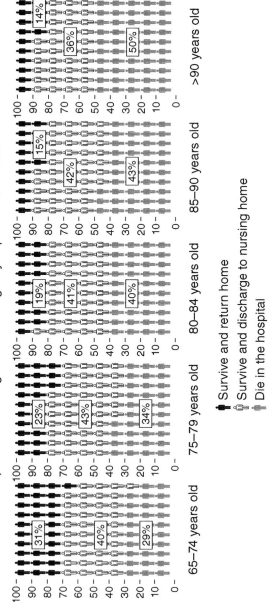

Figure 15.1 Shared decision-making tool for clinicians.

Reproduced from Pallin DJ, et al. Prognosis after emergency department intubation to inform shared decision-making. *J Am Geriatr Soc*, Vol 66(7), 2018, with permission from John Wiley and Sons[24]

In a time-pressured and stressful situation, multiple open-ended questions about the patient's life and wishes may not be informative. Establishing explicit decisions can help the physician to identify salient preferences with regard to the specific situation at hand, rather than broader goals. Once focused on the relevant questions, it may be helpful to guide the conversation with questions like, "What matters to you?", to inform recommendations that would hew with stated priorities. A summary of the plan helps to set expectations for next steps and importantly for future conversations with providers.

15.7 Conclusions

Looking down at a sick patient requiring stabilization, the thought of engaging in the nuanced communication required for shared decision-making can be challenging. EPs should focus on a short list of things to communicate with a patient or their decision maker. Priorities include both the most pressing issues – e.g., confirming prior advance directives – but also setting the stage for future conversations. The role of the EP may not be to subsume more expansive discussions of goals of care but rather to set the precedent that these conversations will happen – that the patient has a voice and that the family can feel empowered to make autonomous choices.

References

1. K.N. Yadav, N.B. Gabler, E. Cooney, et al. Approximately one in three US adults completes any type of advance directive for end-of-life care. *Health Affairs (Millwood)*, 2017; 36(7): 1244–51.

2. S. Wynn. Decisions by surrogates. An overview of surrogate consent laws in the United States. Available: www.americanbar.org/content/dam/aba/publications/bifocal/BIFOCALSeptember-October2014.pdf

3. J.R. Curtis, M.R. Tonelli. Shared decision-making in the ICU: value, challenges, and limitations. *American Journal of Respiratory and Critical Care Medicine*, 2011; 183 (7): 840–1.

4. W.G. Anderson, R.M. Arnold, D.C. Angus, et al. Passive decision-making preference is associated with anxiety and depression in relatives of patients in the intensive care unit. *Journal of Critical Care*, 2009; 24(2): 249–54.

5. K.J. Becker, A.B. Baxter, W.A. Cohen, et al. Withdrawal of support in intracerebral hemorrhage may lead to self-fulfilling prophecies. *Neurology*, 2001; 56: 766–72.

6. A.K. Pratt, J.J. Chang, N.O. Sederstrom. A fate worse than death: prognostication of devastating brain injury. *Critical Care Medicine*, 2019; 47: 591–8.

7. M.J. Souter, P.A. Blissitt, S. Blosser, et al. Recommendations for the critical care management of devastating brain injury: prognostication, psychosocial, and ethical management. *Neurocritical Care*, 2015; 23(1): 4–13.

8. C.J. Creutzfeldt, R.G. Holloway. Treatment decisions for a future self: ethical obligations to guide truly informed choices. *JAMA*, 2020; 323(2): 115–6.

9. G.L. Albrecht, P.J. Devlieger. The disability paradox: high quality of life against all odds. *Social Science and Medicine*, 1999; 48: 977–88.

10. J.C. Hemphill, D.B. White. Clinical nihilism in neuroemergencies. *Emergency Medicine Clinics of North America*, 2009; 27(1): 27–37.

11. M.J. Silveira, W. Wiitala, J. Piette. Advance directive completion by elderly Americans: a decade of change. *Journal of the American Geriatrics Society*, 2014; 62(4): 706–10.

12. S.L. Pedraza, S. Culp, E.C. Falkenstine, et al. POST forms more than advance directives associated with out-of-hospital death: insights from a state registry. *Journal of Pain and Symptom Management*, 2016; 51(2): 240–6.

13. D.K. Richardson, E. Fromme, D. Zive, et al. Concordance of out-of-hospital and emergency department cardiac arrest resuscitation with documented end-of-life choices in Oregon. *Annals of Emergency Medicine*, 2014; 63(4): 375–83.

14. J.L. Chen, J. Sosnov, D. Lessard, et al. Impact of do-not-resuscitation orders on quality of care performance measures in patients hospitalized with acute heart failure. *American Heart Journal*, 2008; 156(1): 78–84.

15. E.A. Jackson, J.L. Yarzebski, R.J. Goldberg, et al. Do-not-resuscitate orders in patients hospitalized with acute myocardial infarction: the Worcester Heart Attack Study. *Archives of Internal Medicine*, 2004; 164(7): 776–83.

16. S.E. Hickman, B.J. Hammes, A.M. Torke, et al. The quality of physician orders for life-sustaining treatment decisions: a pilot study. *Journal of Palliative Medicine*, 2017; 20: 155–62.

17. F.L. Mirarchi, K. Juhasz, T.E. Cooney, et al. TRIAD XII: are patients aware of and agree with DNR or POLST orders in their medical records. *Journal of Patient Safety*, 2019; 15(3): 230–7.

18. G.E. Holt, B. Sarmento, D. Kett, K.W. Goldman. An unconscious patient with a DNR tattoo. *New England Journal of Medicine*, 2017; 377(22): 2192–3.

19. T.I. Cochrane. Unnecessary time pressure in refusal of life-sustaining therapies: dear of missing the opportunity to die. *American Journal of Bioethics*, 2009; 9(4): 47–54.

20. S. Vedantam. The ventilator: life, death and the choices we make at the end. Hidden Brain. NPR; 2019 Nov 19. Available: www.npr.org/2019/11/13/778933239/the-ventilator-life-death-and-the-choices-we-make-at-the-end. (Accessed January 16, 2020.)

21. E.M. Schoenfeld, M.A. Probst, D.D. Quigley, et al. Does shared decision making actually occur in the emergency department? Looking at it from the patient's perspective. *Academic Emergency Medicine*, 2019; 26: 1369–78.

22. I. Hargraves, V.M. Montori. Decision aids, empowerment, and shared decision making. *BMJ*, 2014; 349: g5811.

23. R.T. Griffey, C.D. McNaughton, D.M. McCarthy, et al. Shared decision making in the emergency department among patients with limited health literacy: beyond slower and louder. *Academic Emergency Medicine*, 2016; 23(12): 1403–9.

24. K. Ouchi, G.D. Jambaulikar, S. Hohmann, et al. Prognosis after emergency department intubation to inform shared decision-making. *Journal of the American Geriatrics Society*, 2018; 66(7): 1377–81.

Advance Directives

Law, Policy, and Use in Shared
Decision-Making

16

Joshua Rolnick

Advance directives (ADs) are legal documents that provide information on a patient's preferences for care when seriously ill. ADs include two separate documents: a health-care power of attorney and/or a living will. This Chapter provides a practical guide to questions that may arise in the use of ADs as a part of shared decision-making in the intensive care unit (ICU).

A living will documents a patient's wishes for health-care at the end of life. For all its limitations, the living will may be the ICU practitioner's only direct record of a patient's wishes. Documentation in the medical record, although important, is indirect, created by a clinician as a record of conversations with a patient and their family.

A durable health-care power of attorney is a legal document that designates an individual or individuals to make health care decisions when a patient lacks capacity for decision-making. It is called "durable" because it remains in effect even when the patient lacks capacity, in contrast to a standard financial power of attorney. Usually, a health care agent has the authority to make all or nearly all decisions that a patient would be able to make. The agent's authority supersedes that of closer family members. Even when the agent is not related to the patient, or does not speak the ICU practitioner's language, it is the agent, not closer family members, who have legal decision-making authority.

16.1 Legal Questions

What law governs ADs? In the United States, ADs are usually governed by state law, with some exceptions for the Veterans Health Administration and the Department of Defense.[1] Rules for legal formalities, when ADs take legal effect, and other important issues will vary. When ICU practitioners move from one state to another, they should be aware that these legal factors may change.[2,3]

What does it mean that an AD is "legally binding?" When a living will or health-care power of attorney takes effect, it means that clinicians are obligated to follow the wishes of the document in designating a decision-maker or specifying wishes for care. In return, most jurisdictions establish a legal safe harbor, immunizing clinicians from criminal, civil, or administrative (e.g., medical board) action for good faith efforts to follow an AD. In reality, for living wills, clinicians have an "out" if they disagree with the wishes for care, usually by transferring the patient, leading some commentators to describe living wills as "legally recognized" rather than "legally binding."[4]

When do these documents take effect legally? Although living wills and health-care power of attorney documents are bundled together as ADs, they take effect in different circumstances. A durable health-care power of attorney takes effect when the patient lacks capacity to make medical decisions – a legal status known as incompetence – regardless of the patient's medical prognosis. For example, in Pennsylvania, the law states that a health-care power of attorney takes effect when (1) a copy is provided to the attending physician and (2) the attending physician determines that the patient lacks capacity.[5] However, the health-care power of attorney documentation can specify different circumstances.

In contrast, a living will does *not* take effect whenever the patient is incompetent. In most states, the patient must also be near the end of life. Pennsylvania, for example, requires that the patient have an end-stage medical condition or be permanently unconscious. An end-stage medical condition is an "incurable and irreversible medical condition" that would "result in death" despite full treatment measures.[6] Conditions that may, to an ICU practitioner, be reasonable circumstances in which some patients and families may wish to avoid aggressive treatment measures – an older, frail patient with mild dementia requiring intubation to treat pneumonia – may not meet the requirements for a living will to take effect, even though the health-care power of attorney is in effect. That agent, however, is still required under the law of most states to exercise substituted judgment whenever possible, meaning to make the decisions they believe the patient would have wanted. An "inoperative" living will may still clinically be a useful tool in understanding patient wishes and facilitating conversations with family members.

Are ADs from one state valid to use in another state? The validity of an AD from a different state, or country, will depend on local law. U.S. states follow two models: (1) some recognize an out-of-state AD as valid only if it meets legal formalities in the local jurisdiction where the patient is hospitalized, whereas (2) other states recognize an out-of-state AD, even if not adherent to local standards, provided it meets the requirements of the jurisdiction in which it was created.[4]

Who makes decisions if a patient has no health-care power of attorney? Nearly every jurisdiction has rules for default surrogate status. The most common order of priority is spouse, adult child, parent, adult sibling, adult grandchild, and close friend, with the specifics varying by jurisdiction.

The default rules are often indeterminate – if the patient has more than one adult child, those children will have equal decision-making status. Laws may specify that if health-care representatives do not agree, the attending physician may rely on a consensus view of a majority of the surrogates who have communicated their perspectives.

Clinicians often treat nonagent decision-makers the same as agents, assuming they have equal authority to make decisions. In fact, such is not the case in all jurisdictions – at least as a matter of technical legal fact – and nonagents may lack the same decision-making authority as agents. In Pennsylvania, for example, nonagents cannot withdraw life-prolonging measures unless the patient has an end-stage medical condition, leaving a gray zone of medical circumstances in which aggressive interventions such as mechanical ventilation may not be consistent with patient wishes, yet not technically permissible to withhold from incompetent patients under the law.[7]

What should happen if a family disagrees with the wishes in a living will? Under the law, if a living will is operative and speaks clearly to the clinical issue, it will almost always supersede the wishes of the family, even a family member appointed as an agent. In practice, such conflicts are challenging to navigate. Clinicians may feel ethically obligated to respect patient wishes. They may also worry about worsening bereavement on the part of families, who may dispute that the living will accurately reflect patient wishes. In the ideal scenario, such disputes would be prevented in advance, through clear communication between patient and family about the wishes a patient plans to document. The living will's communication function may be useful in these situations; clinicians should engage fully with families and try to understand if legal documentation and family wishes can be reconciled.

What happens if family members disagree with the health-care agent? Under the law, the health-care agent – even if not physically present, not related to the patient, or unable to communicate with clinicians without an interpreter – has legal authority to make decisions. But a health-care agent may wish to engage other family members in the decision-making process, or, at a minimum, allow them to remain informed about the patient's medical status.

Health-care agents have duties in both statutes and common law (judge-made law) to use certain principles to make decisions. Generally, they are expected to exercise substituted judgment, meaning to make the decisions they believe the patient would have made in similar circumstances, even though understanding what a patient would want may be challenging in many circumstances. When patient wishes cannot be known, then they revert to a best interest standard, one that makes the decision that relies on community norms.

Are pregnant patients treated differently? In some states, they are treated differently, and may be limited in withdrawing care, even through a living will or the decisions of a duly appointed health-care agent.[8]

Are digital ADs legally binding? Websites such "mydirectives" offer the ability to create electronic ADs. The legal status of digitally signing an AD is still unclear, except in specific jurisdictions (e.g., Maryland and California). Whether legally binding or not, however, digital living wills may still serve the communication function of living wills.

16.2 Clinical Questions

What is the evidence of the impact of ADs on end-of-life care? The evidence is mixed. Observational studies have shown an association between having ADs and avoiding high-intensity care.[9–11] However, the potential for confounding is high in these studies, because AD completion may be associated with personal qualities affecting end-of-life decisions, qualities not easily captured by measured variables from either claims or electronic health records. Experimental evidence has been less consistent, often finding little relationship between ADs and outcomes that may matter for end-of-life care, such as lower intensity care or less preference-discordant care.[12–14]

One challenge in these studies is the highly contextual effect of ADs. The document itself may matter less than the communication process underlying its creation. The AD may represent an advance care planning process that included AD completion. However, that process may vary extensively. It may have involved completing documents with a lawyer in isolation, without clear communication with clinicians or family. Or it may have involved in-depth conversations leading in part to the creation of legal documents. The impact of the AD may only be as good as the process that produced it.

What are the barriers to use of ADs to improve end-of-life decision-making? ADs could improve decision-making in two respects. First, they could improve decision-making for patients, by increasing the likelihood of receiving care consistent with preferences and values. Second, they could improve decision-making for family members and caregivers, by reducing decisional distress. ADs face several barriers to accomplishing these goals. First, they are rarely completed.[15] Second, when completed, they are often unavailable in the electronic health record, for ICU practitioners and other clinicians to use when decisions must be made.[16] Third, the content is often unhelpful in guiding decision-making, and living wills did not improve surrogate-patient decision concordance in one randomized study.[9]

How then should ICU practitioners most effectively use ADs? Practitioners should first distinguish between the two components of an AD, the health-care power of attorney and the living will. ICU practitioners should remember that legally appointed health-care agents have decision-making priority over closer family members. That decision-making ability should be respected except in specific circumstances. However, relying on an agent does not necessarily mean ignoring other people close to the patient, and other family members may be involved in discussions about patient care as deemed appropriate by the agent and encouraged by clinicians.

Living wills function primarily as communication tools, rather than legal documents, in most clinical circumstances.[17] Often, they do not directly address a clinical scenario, either because preconditions are not met (e.g., the patient is not end stage or permanently unconscious) or because they do not address the specific clinical decision that must be made. However, they may help offer some guidance as to patient wishes, or at least help to prompt discussions with family members. Clinicians may wish to ask about family involvement in creating an AD and what conversations about wishes occurred during that process.

What steps would make ADs more useful as a tool for shared decision-making? Planning for ADs – not just the act of creating legal paperwork! – helps prepare patients and families for decision-making.[18] ADs are best viewed as a component of a larger process in which patients discuss their wishes with family members, other loved ones, and clinicians. Patients should ensure that their chosen surrogates know they have been designated as legal agents, and discuss their wishes with those agents. When patients survive intensive care and regain their ability to make decisions, ICU practitioners may wish to encourage them to complete ADs, and do so as part of a larger process of advance care planning that includes family members and clinicians.

References

1. Policy and Guidance - National Center for Ethics in Health Care. Available: www.ethics.va.gov/policy.asp#Advance%20Care%20Planning%20and%20Management%20of%20Advance%20Directives. (Accessed January 1, 2020).

2. L.S. Castillo, B.A. Williams, S.M. Hooper, et al. Lost in translation: The unintended consequences of advance directive law on clinical care. *Annals of Internal Medicine*, 2011; 154(2): 121–8.

3. E.S. DeMartino, J.A. Rolnick. The states as laboratories: regulation of decisions for incapacitated patients. *Journal of Clinical Ethics*, 2019; 30(2): 89–95.

4. Can my advance directives travel across state lines? An essay on portability. Available: www.americanbar.org/groups/law_aging/publications/bifocal/vol_38/issue_1_october2016/advance-directives-across-state-lines/. (Accessed January 1, 2020).

5. *20 Pa.C.S. § 5454(a) (2017).*

6. *20 Pa.C.S. § 5422 (2017).*

7. *In Re D.L.H., 606 Pa. 550, 2 A.3d 505 (2010).*

8. E.S. DeMartino, B.P. Sperry, C.K. Doyle, et al. US state regulation of decisions for pregnant women without decisional capacity. *JAMA*, 2019; 321(16): 1629.

9. J.M. Teno, A. Gruneir, Z. Schwartz, et al. Association between advance directives and quality of end-of-life care: a national study: Advance directives and the quality of end-of-life care. *Journal of the American Geriatrics Society*, 2007; 55(2): 189–94.

10. M.J. Silveira, S.Y.H. Kim, K.M. Langa. Advance directives and outcomes of surrogate decision making before death. *New England Journal of Medicine*, 2010; 362(13): 1211–18.

11. L.H. Nicholas, K.M. Langa, T.J. Iwashyna, et al. Regional variation in the association between advance directives and end-of-life Medicare expenditures. *JAMA*, 2011; 306 (13): 1447–53.

12. P.H. Ditto, J.H. Danks, W.D. Smucker, et al. Advance directives as acts of communication: a randomized controlled trial. *Archives of Internal Medicine*, 2001; 161(3): 421–30.

13. D.W. Molloy, G.H. Guyatt, R. Russo, et al. Systematic implementation of an advance directive program in nursing homes: a randomized controlled trial. *JAMA*, 2000; 283(11): 1437.

14. K.M. Detering, A.D. Hancock, M.C. Reade, et al. The impact of advance care planning on end of life care in elderly patients: randomised controlled trial. *BMJ*, 2010; 340: c1345.

15. K.N. Yadav, N.B. Gabler, E. Cooney, et al. Approximately one in three US adults completes any type of advance directive for end-of-life care. *Health Affairs (Millwood)*, 2017; 36(7): 1244–51.

16. C.J. Wilson, J. Newman, S. Tapper, et al. Multiple locations of advance care planning documentation in an electronic health record: are they easy to find? *Journal of Palliative Medicine*, 2013; 16(9): 1089–94.

17. C.P. Sabatino. The evolution of health care advance planning law and policy. *Milbank Quarterly*, 2010; 88(2): 211–39.

18. J.A. Rolnick, D.A. Asch, S.D. Halpern. Delegalizing advance directives – facilitating advance care planning. *New England Journal of Medicine*, 2017; 376(22): 2105–7.

Care of the Unbefriended Patient

Stephen Trevick

"Unbefriended," or "unrepresented," patients are those who are unable to make their own decisions with regard to their medical care and lack an available surrogate decision maker. As we discuss in this Chapter, many terms have been used to refer to this heterogeneous group, although none fully encompass the breadth of clinical scenarios that present in critical illness; we use "unbefriended patient" for consistency. This unfortunate situation may occur because the person is truly without close contacts or those contacts are unable to be contacted to make these critical decisions on behalf of the patient. Patients without available surrogates but with clearly documented goals of care have variably been included or excluded from this cohort. Although these scenarios may, at first glance, seem to be at the edges of the management spectrum, they are not uncommon. In two studies, 16% of patients who were admitted to the intensive care unit (ICU) and 5.5% of patients who died in the ICU were without surrogates.[1,2] The care of these individuals strains the legal, ethical, and practical limits of our work and must be explored by both individual physicians and their institutions.

17.1 Complications for the Unbefriended Patient

Unbefriended patients are a vulnerable group and are often members of underrepresented and disabled communities.[3] Autonomy is one of the central principles of medical ethics, and without clear representation or knowledge of a patient's goals, the direction of care cannot accurately reflect their wishes. Therapy may not only lack respect to individualized goals but are also often biased away from palliative care. Patients lacking surrogates have fewer palliative care consults, chaplain visits, and do-not-resuscitate orders than represented patients.[4] They are also found to have longer stays in the ICU than represented patients, but without any conferred improvement in mortality.[1] These factors are a reflection of the various complications presented in the care of the unbefriended patient.

Guidelines from state law, medical administration, and specialty associations are varied and lacking. Providers themselves are often worried about future reprisals or legal culpability when considering palliative approaches to these patients.[5] The lack of a clear surrogate can also produce practical challenges to enrollment in hospice and the attainment of services.

17.2 Guidelines and Resources

United States law values autonomy highly, particularly in relation to end-of-life decision-making. The law is generally designed to respect autonomy and provide for its maintenance in cases where patients have lost the capacity to inform their own care. Its very nature is why patient-designated surrogates, such as individuals with a written power of attorney, are the most highly respected in the order of surrogacy. When wishes are documented, but no surrogate is available to help in their interpretation, the physician may, theoretically, interpret and follow its instruction. However, the guidance provided by these forms is rarely so specifically written or easy to apply in any individual patient's particular case.[6] As such, documented instructions for goals of care are important tools for patient surrogates, but not a substitute for the surrogate altogether.

This situation presents a lacune in the law for unbefriended patients. Some states make allowances, including a law enacted in 2011 by Oregon, that enable hospitals to appoint "a health care provider who has received training in health care ethics" as the patient's surrogate.[7] Other states require the designation of a court-appointed guardian, which is often a time-consuming and cumbersome process.[8] Overall, at least six different models exist surrounding the care of the unbefriended patient in the 13 states with clearly defined laws on the subject.[9] Despite the heterogeneity of state laws on the subject, it is clear that the provider–surrogate dyad is upheld as a vital aspect of autonomy. Simply put, it is presumed that at the very least a representative will be engaged in end-of-life decisions for patients with the treating physician.

The recommendations of professional bodies also demonstrate some heterogeneity. The American Medical Association recommends ethics committee or judicial review, whereas the American College of Physicians recommends only judicial review.[10,11] The American Geriatrics Society (AGS) had advised against routine court involvement, deferring to the individual clinician caring for the patient[12]; however, in 2016 they revised this position suggesting referral to an external entity, such as an ethics committee "when time allows."[13] This revision cited the need for "adequate safeguards" against "physician bias or conflicts of interest."

In one study that identified 37 unbefriended patients for whom a physician considered limiting life support, only six underwent internal institutional review, and one received a judicial review. Among the remaining 30 patients, the treating team did not appeal to outside review, although in 16 of these cases they did consult a second attending physician.[2] The study enrolled patients across seven different hospitals, two of which did not have institution-specific instructions concerning the management of the unbefriended patient. Within the remaining five facilities, one recommended appointing a hospital advocate, one allowed the attending physician to decide unilaterally, two required the review of an ethics committee, and one requested either a second attending or ethics committee review, depending on the specifics of the case. This study serves to highlight, again, the discord between guidelines and the extent to which they are directly followed.

17.3 Variability among Unbefriended Patients

The many terms used, such as the unbefriended patient, the unrepresented patient, or the adult orphan, conjure the image of a wholly abandoned patient left without any means for guidance in their care. There is, however, considerably more variability found within this population. The unbefriended patient is considered a person who lacks capacity and does not have representation through a surrogate or clear advance directives. Advance directives themselves, even when present, may or may not be clear and directly applicable to a given situation. Carefully documented and attested directions for only comfort directed care would be relatively easy to implement, however, statements such as not wanting to be kept alive if "severely disabled," although common, are often much harder to interpret. Therefore, patients with advance directives but no designated surrogate are often included among the grouping of unbefriended patients, although clearly with an important, if not independently sufficient, guide to their care.

The unbefriended patient lacks capacity. However, capacity, in its medical sense, is time and question specific.[8] Therefore, a patient may have fluctuating capacity, particularly in the ICU setting. Furthermore, a patient may have capacity for some decisions and not others.[14] Capacity requires an understanding of the salient features of the decision, the ability to express a choice, an appreciation of the impact of the choice, and reasoning to come to a decision.[15] A patient may have the capacity to name a surrogate, but lack the ability to fully understand the impact of a complex surgery or medical intervention. Importantly, when patients do not have the capacity to make a medical decision, they may still be able to report overall desires and goals, such as long-held values toward quantity or quality of life, or, lacking this, express their current experience and level of suffering. This can provide vital guidance for care, without rising to the level of decisional capacity.[16]

Although some patients may be without identifiable contacts of any sort, others may have friends and family but not formal surrogates for one reason or another. Some contacts may be unwilling to take on the responsibility and burden of making these sorts of decisions for patients, whereas others may have some knowledge or acquaintance with the patient but insufficient to help direct care. Patient contacts may have their own medical or other practical factors limiting their ability to engage in detailed discussion, or they may lack capacity themselves. Clinicians are obligated to assess the capacity of a surrogate much as they would for a patient, although possibly with a more limited knowledge of their current medical state. If a patient contact (or contacts) is discovered who cannot rise to the level of surrogate, the patient may remain technically "unbefriended," but with a new source of information to assist in the decision-making process.

17.4 Approaches and Considerations in the Care of the Unbefriended Patient

Clearly, the unbefriended patient is in an undesirable state, and thus the first and foremost approach must be prevention. When a patient without an identified surrogate arrives in the ICU, one should be identified as quickly as possible. Capacity can shift quickly, and someone who enters the ICU making their own decisions may quickly lose that ability. As discussed, patients without capacity to make all their medical decisions may retain the capacity to name a surrogate, provide useful collateral sources of information, and express values and goals, which may all be helpful in rendering future decisions. This provides yet another reason to address goals of care early in the hospital or ICU course.

When searching for a surrogate decision maker, nontraditional options may be of use. The exact hierarchy of surrogate decision makers varies by state, but generally follows the designated power-of-attorney, spouse, first-degree relative, distant relative, then close friend. This last category can be quite flexible and may include any person with knowledge of the patient's goals who has the patient's interests at heart and agrees to the position of surrogate. Many hospitals require a written or even notarized affidavit to this effect. Depending on the situation, a "close-friend surrogate" may be a neighbor, nonmarried partner, fellow member of a religious institution, or even a professional contact such as a physician or lawyer. In these less common situations, care must be provided to ensure the absence of conflicts of interest. Legal statutes may exclude certain groups, such as providers linked to active care, although these too vary by state.[16] When this is unclear, an ethics consultant or risk specialist may be of assistance.

Some individual contacts of patients may be unavailable to engage in sufficient conversation with the care team to help guide decisions. Some may have cognitive deficits limiting their appropriateness and capacity to take on the decision-making role. Others may simply not desire to act as the decision maker. These contacts can help to provide useful information about the patient's prior state of health, lifestyle, and wishes as well, even if not rising to the role of substitute decision makers.

Many decisions must be made in the care of any patient in the ICU and are often more emergent than previously described investigations to find surrogate decisions makers among contacts may allow. Emergency or "two-physician" consent may cover immediate decision-making concerns. However, although the specific wording of this clause varies from state to state, it assumes a continued, good faith effort by the medical team to find a surrogate. Thus, necessary medical treatment may continue in parallel to exploring the other decision-making avenues described here.

As explained, recommendations vary between professional societies; however, all recommend a patient's surrogate to be separate from the treatment team to best respect the patient's autonomy and avoid bias. Institutional review boards – generally ethics committees – can act in this capacity, as the American Medical Association and AGS recommend. Ethics committees and consultants can also aid in the discovery of surrogates and collateral information regarding a patient's wishes, although these resources can vary greatly in availability and scale between institutions.

In cases where no personal surrogate may be found, one may be appointed by a governmental agency. The laws and resources for this, again, vary state by state. Although some states make provisions for the temporary appointment of guardians in emergent situations, generally this process is somewhat prolonged and cumbersome and may require several weeks. The appointed guardian should weigh whatever information is available about the patient's wishes and act to best represent their interests. Of course, these guardians are without personal knowledge of the patient and are often overburdened with cases. They are often necessary for certain placements outside of the hospital, implementation of services, and decisions such as the withdrawal of life support.

Cases of severe illness in unbefriended patients are difficult and benefit from marshalling all resources available. Early involvement of ethics consultants or committees and risk management can help to guide care and identify possible alternate surrogates or sources of information. They can also help to provide guidance as to local legal precedents and institutional policies.

17.5 Progress and Future Directions

Care of the unbefriended patient requires the guidance and resources of legislatures and hospitals. In fact, five of the nine recommendations of the 2016 AGS statement on the care of the unbefriended patient address healthcare systems. These include making it easier and more common for patients to express their own directives in easily actionable forms before the loss of capacity to make decisions for themselves and creating more standardized pathways for the care of unbefriended patients. Provider Orders for Life-Sustaining Treatment are being used in more and more states, thereby allowing simple, durable, and transferrable advance directives. Advance directives, in all their forms, can help to ameliorate the loss of autonomy a patient suffers without decisional capacity or surrogates.

Increased national standardization on the part of professional organizations is helpful, although legal standards generally fall to the state. Two main avenues have been used to improve the care of unbefriended patients: standardizing and expanding the list of possible surrogates to include close friends or additional nontraditional options as well as improving the process to obtain public guardianship. Some states have worked to speed the process of guardianship in emergent situations and overall improve resources available to these programs.[17,18]

Hospitals must provide support to clinicians caring for unbefriended patients. This may be done through the development of clinical policies to help standardize care and education surrounding policies, available resources, and state laws. Risk management and ethics committees are valuable resources and make excellent avenues through which clinicians may become involved and improve the care of these most vulnerable patients.

References

1. D.B. White, J.R. Curtis, B. Lo, et al. Decisions to limit life sustaining treatment for critically ill patients who lack both decision-making capacity and surrogate decision-makers. *Critical Care Medicine*, 2006; 34(8): 2053–9.

2. D.B. White, J.R. Curtis, L.E. Wolf, et al. Life support for patients without a surrogate decision maker: who decides? *Annals of Internal Medicine*, 2007; 147(1): 34–40.

3. H. Kim, M.K. Song. Medical decision-making for adults who lack decision-making capacity and a surrogate: state of the science. *Journal of Hospice and Palliative Care* 2018; 35(9): 1227.

4. R.L. Sudore, D. Casarett, D. Smith, et al. Family involvement at the end-of-life and receipt of quality care. *Journal of Pain and Symptom Management*, 2014; 48(6): 1108–16.

5. A. Effiong, S. Harman. Patients who lack capacity and lack surrogates: can they enroll in hospice? *Journal of Pain and Symptom Management*, 2014; 48(4): 745–50.

6. N. Karp, E. Wood. Incapacitated and alone: healthcare decision making for unbefriended older people. *Human Rights*, 2004; 31(2): 20–4.

7. Oregon S.B. 579, 76th Legis. Assembly (2011), enacted Ch. 512, 2011 Laws.

8. T.M. Pope. Legal fundamentals of surrogate decision making. *Chest*, 2012; 141(4): 1074–81.

9. D. Godfrey. *Health care decision making during a crisis when nothing is in writing.* Vienna, VA: National Academy of Elder Law Attorneys; 2019.

10. American Medical Association, Council on Ethical and Judicial Affairs. *Code of medical ethics, current opinions with annotations: Including the principles of medical ethics, fundamental elements of the patient-physician relationship and rules of the council on ethical and judicial affairs.* Chicago: American Medical Association; 2004.

11. L. Snyder, C. Leffler. Ethics and Human Rights Committee, American College of Physicians. Ethics manual, fifth edition. *Annals of Internal Medicine*, 2005; 142: 560–82.

12. AGS Ethics Committee. Making treatment decisions for incapacitated older adults without advance directives. *Journal of the American Geriatrics Society*, 1996; 44: 986–7.

13. T.W. Farrell, E. Widera, L. Rosenberg, et al. AGS position statement: making medical treatment decisions for unbefriended older adults. *Journal of the American Geriatrics Society*, 2017; 65(1): 14–15.

14. P.S. Appelbaum. Clinical practice. Assessment of patients' competence to consent to treatment. *New England Journal of Medicine*, 2007; 357(18): 1834.

15. T. Grisso, P.S. Appelbaum. Abilities related to competence. In: *Assessing competence to consent to treatment: A guide for physicians and other health professionals.* New York: Oxford University Press; 1998; pp. 31.

16. T.M. Pope, T. Sellers. Legal briefing: the unbefriended: Making healthcare decisions for patients without surrogates (part 1). *Journal of Clinical Ethics*, 2012; 23(1): 84–96.

17. T.M. Pope. Unbefriended and unrepresented: medical decision making for incapacitated patients without healthcare surrogates. *Georgia State University Law Review*, 2017; 33(4): pp. 923–1019.

18. T.M. Pope. Legal briefing: Adult orphans and the unbefriended: making medical decisions for unrepresented patients without surrogates. *Journal of Clinical Ethics*, 2015; 26(2): 180–8.

The Role of Palliative Care in the Intensive Care Unit

Adeline L. Goss and Claire J. Creutzfeldt

18.1 Defining Palliative Care

Originating mostly in the world of oncology, palliative care has matured into a wide-ranging field aimed at improving the quality of life of all patients and their families facing the problems associated with life-threatening illnesses. Palliative care aims at preventing and relieving physical, social, psychological, and spiritual suffering. Components of palliative care vary based on the setting, but generally include (1) relationship and rapport building with patients and family members; (2) addressing and managing physical, social, psychological, and spiritual symptoms; (3) eliciting patient and family values; (4) interpreting and communicating information about the patient's illness, prognosis, and treatment options and ensuring understanding; (5) helping patients and families to cope with life-altering circumstances and preventing or managing grief; (6) identifying and resolving conflicts, either between family members, between different medical team members, or between family and medical teams; (7) assisting with goal setting and advance care planning; and (8) hospice referral and discharge planning.[1,2] Palliative care can be provided to patients and their families in any setting and at any time during the course of an illness, and may be offered alongside curative treatment.

Palliative care needs in the intensive care unit (ICU) setting are substantial. Not only does one in five Americans die in the ICU,[3] but survivors of critical illness report a high symptom burden, including pain, difficulty communicating, dyspnea, hunger, and confusion.[4,5] After ICU discharge, patients continue to have higher rates of mortality and may suffer from functional limitations and poor health-related quality of life.[6–8] Patients often lack the capacity to participate in medical decision-making, requiring the involvement of surrogate decision makers, who may have their own palliative care needs. These individuals have a high burden of adverse psychological outcomes even long after the ICU stay, owing to the burden of decision-making, caregiving, and complicated grief. As a result of all of these factors, efforts to integrate high-quality palliative care into intensive care have the potential to benefit all ICU patients and their families.

18.2 Primary and Specialist Palliative Care

The framework of the palliative care approach describes the care that patients and their families receive, rather than the clinician or team providing this care. This approach aims to ensure that patients receive palliative care as they need it, across a wide range of settings, including the home, outpatient, inpatient, and hospice settings. It is based on the idea that palliative care, like any subspecialty, includes certain skills that all health-care providers should possess as well as more specialized skills that require dedicated training.

The palliative care approach encompasses what are often referred to as "primary" and "specialist" palliative care. "Primary palliative care" is that provided by the primary medical team (i.e., the intensivist for a patient hospitalized with acute respiratory distress syndrome). These are the providers leading the patient's medical care and providing the patient and their family with medical information about the patient's present illness, prognosis, and available treatment options. The primary team is responsible for the identification of palliative care needs and basic management of distressing symptoms. In most cases, the primary team should also take the lead on shared decision-making: ensuring illness understanding, eliciting the patient's treatment preferences and values, and recommending courses of treatment tailored to those preferences and values – or, in the case of patients who lack decision-making capacity, supporting surrogates to provide substituted judgment. Table 18.1 provides a list of these and other primary palliative care skills.

In ICU settings, palliative care may also be provided by palliative care specialists in the role of a consulting team, which typically includes physicians and advanced practice registered nurses and may also include social workers, chaplains, physician assistants, nurses, pharmacists, and/or psychologists.[10] Palliative care consultants are often called upon by the primary team in cases of uncontrolled symptom distress, for conflict resolution and mediation, for assistance with particularly complex goals-of-care discussions, or when planning transitions of care.

The availability of palliative care services in the United States continues to grow. As of 2016–2017, according to the Center to Advance Palliative Care's 2019 report card, palliative care programs (broadly defined) were available in 72% of U.S. hospitals with 50 or more beds. Significant regional variation persists, however, i.e., only 17% of rural hospitals with 50 or more beds reported having palliative care programs.[11]

18.3 Models of Palliative Care Involvement in the ICU

Efforts to integrate palliative care into intensive care may be classified as consultative and integrative models. Consultative models bring palliative care

Table 18.1. Primary palliative care skills

Pain and symptoms

Recognize early signs of pain, anxiety, delirium, etc.

Basic symptom management skills

Communication skills

Communicate with empathy and compassion

Listen actively and attentively

Practice narrative competence to elicit the patient's story

Elicit the patient's values and treatment preferences (see Goals of care)

Share information with the patient and family using terms they understand

Communicate prognosis for quantity and quality of life

Provide anticipatory guidance regarding illness and treatment trajectories

Develop consensus for difficult decisions in a manner that is sensitive to the patient's/family's preferred role of decision-making

Identify and manage moral distress among interdisciplinary team members

Psychosocial and spiritual support

Identify psychosocial and emotional needs of patients and families

Identify needs for spiritual or religious support and provide referrals

Access resources that can help to meet psychosocial needs

Practice cultural humility

Goals of care

Help to establish goals of care based on patient values, goals, and treatment preferences, or through substituted judgment

Engage in shared decision-making and adapt shared decision-making approaches to patient and family preferences

Incorporate ethical principles in communication and decision-making

End-of-life issues

Emphasize non-abandonment and provide continued emotional support through the dying process for patients and their families

Provide anticipatory guidance regarding the dying process

Facilitate bereavement support for family members

Basic palliative care skills that all ICU physicians should master. Adapted with permission from Creutzfeldt et al., 2015[9]

consultants into the ICU to interact with patients and family members. Integrative models embed palliative care principles and interventions into daily ICU practice, but only ICU personnel interact with patients and families. Many of these interventions have been evaluated in the ICU setting.[12,13] These two types of models are not mutually exclusive, and a mix of the two is common in clinical practice.

18.4 Consultative and Integrative Models

Consultative models provide palliative care services to select ICU patients, and their effectiveness has been fairly well-studied. A series of before–after, single-center trials of such consultative models have suggested an association between palliative care consultation with decreased ICU length of stay,[14–18] lower hospital costs,[19] earlier initiation of do-not-resuscitate orders and withdrawal of life support,[17] and increased family satisfaction with the hospital experience and decision-making process,[20] with no difference in hospital length of stay, length of stay from ICU admission to discharge, or mortality.[14,17,18]

In many so-called integrative models, critical care teams incorporate palliative care principles and interventions for all patients and families in the ICU.[12] A substantial source of stress among family members of critically ill patients is the burden of surrogate decision-making, which may be measured as symptoms of anxiety, depression, and post-traumatic stress disorder. Many integrative models aim to improve communication between ICU providers and families, providing both emotional and informational support to surrogates as they navigate treatment decisions. For example, providing family members with printed informational brochures and decision aids has been shown to improve their comprehension.[21,22] Connecting family members with specialists trained to facilitate communication (such as social workers or ICU nurses) has been associated with higher rates of do-not-resuscitate/do-not-intubate and comfort care only status, as well as higher rates of decisions to treat the patient aggressively,[23] suggesting that the intervention, importantly, served to clarify treatment preferences. Communication facilitators have also been associated with higher physician and surrogate ratings of communication,[24,25] decreased depressive symptoms at 6 months, lower ICU costs,[26] and decreased ICU length of stay.[25,26] One study found increased rates of hospital death but no difference in death at 6 months.[25] An alternative integrative approach focuses on standardizing family meetings. Standardizing the meeting structure has been associated with reduced family member post-traumatic stress disorder,[27] while ensuring that family meetings occur within 72 hours of ICU admission has been associated with decreased mortality, decreased ICU length of stay, and fewer days when there was disagreement on the long-term disposition goal between ICU providers and between ICU providers and families.[28,29] Other integrative interventions include palliative care-related clinician education, family presence on rounds, and standardized palliative care-related order sets.[12]

A systematic review comparing consultative to integrative models of palliative care interventions in the ICU found insufficient evidence to favor one approach over the other.[12] Both models have potential disadvantages. Implementation of an integrative model requires ICU teams to take on extra duties, which may be particularly challenging in open ICU models, where many providers of different specialties would require training on a given intervention. Consultative models, meanwhile, require hiring and training of new personnel, which may not be feasible at many centers.[12] Additionally, some have raised concerns that excessive reliance on specialist palliative care could fragment care; undermine existing therapeutic relationships between primary providers, patients, and families; and decrease incentives for primary providers to develop palliative care skills.[30]

18.5 Palliative Care Triggers

Another approach to palliative care consultation in the ICU relies on critical care teams meeting basic palliative care needs while employing "trigger" systems or checklists to involve palliative care consultants for more complex cases. Trigger systems involve palliative care consultants in prespecified clinical scenarios (Table 18.2), and have been shown to increase rates of palliative care consultations.[14,31,32]

Trigger systems identify patients at high risk for palliative care needs, but do not provide a means for ICU teams to assess those needs. An alternative model uses checklists on daily ICU rounds that both screen for palliative care needs that can be met by the primary team and aid in recognizing the need for involvement of palliative care specialists. In the chapter authors' field of neurology, critically ill patients are often at risk of early mortality, but also have the potential for considerable recovery. Among those who survive, there may be significant disability and symptom burden. Despite this, patients with acute severe neurologic disease infrequently receive palliative care services.[33,34] Structured screening programs can help to meet the palliative care needs of this population; in one study, the use of a four-question palliative care needs checklist on ICU rounds was associated with more documented family meetings.[35]

18.6 Conclusions

Palliative care is an integrated field that works in conjunction with other medical specialties to improve quality of life and ameliorate symptom burden in any life-threatening disease, regardless of diagnosis, prognosis, or setting.

Table 18.2. Some proposed palliative care triggers[14,31,32]

Hospitalization characteristics
Prolonged ICU admission (e.g., >10 days; >1 month)
More than three ICU admissions during the present hospitalization
Exceeding length of stay by >50%
Patient characteristics
Advanced age (e.g., >70 or 80 years of age) with multiple life-threatening comorbidities
Specific diagnoses
Diagnosis of active metastatic malignancy
Intracerebral hemorrhage with mechanical ventilation
Various Glasgow Coma Scale cutoffs (e.g., Glasgow Coma Score of <8 for >1week in a patient >75 years old; Glasgow Coma Score of 3)
Multiorgan failure
Specific prognoses
Futility considered or declared by the medical team
Death expected during the ICU stay
Family factors
Family request
Family disagreement with the medical team, advance directive, or each other for >7 days
Family experiencing severe distress
Family displaying worrisome coping skills such as denial or ambivalence
Family needing extended periods of time to explore goals and values

A wide variety of models has been suggested for integrating palliative care into the critical care setting, and more research is needed to define the role of both primary and specialist palliative care in the ICU. Improving access to both primary and specialist palliative care has the potential to benefit all ICU patients and their families.

References

1. L.N. Tran, A.L. Back, C.J. Creutzfeldt. Palliative care consultations in the neuro-ICU: a qualitative study. *Neurocritical Care*, 2016; 25(2): 266–72.

2. J. Yoong, E.R. Park, J.A. Greer, et al. Early palliative care in advanced lung cancer: a qualitative study. *JAMA Internal Medicine*, 2013; 173(4): 283–90.

3. D.C. Angus, A.E. Barnato, W.T. Linde-Zwirble, et al. Use of intensive care at the end of life in the United States: an epidemiologic study. *Critical Care Medicine*, 2004; 32(3): 638–43.

4. J.E. Nelson, D.E. Meier, A. Litke, et al. The symptom burden of chronic critical illness. *Critical Care Medicine*, 2004; 32(7): 1527–34.

5. K.A. Puntillo, S. Arai, N.H. Cohen, , et al. Symptoms experienced by intensive care unit patients at high risk of dying. *Critical Care Medicine*, 2010; 38(11): 2155–60.

6. C.E. Cox, S.S. Carson, J.H. Lindquist, et al. Differences in one-year health outcomes and resource utilization by definition of prolonged mechanical ventilation: a prospective cohort study. *Critical Care*, 2007; 11(1): R9.

7. C.E. Cox, S.L. Docherty, D.H. Brandon, et al. Surviving critical illness: acute respiratory distress syndrome as experienced by patients and their caregivers. *Critical Care Medicine*, 2009; 37(10): 2702–8.

8. H. Wunsch, C. Guerra, A.E. Barnato, et al. Three-year outcomes for medicare beneficiaries who survive intensive care. *JAMA*, 2010; 303(9): 849–56.

9. C.J. Creutzfeldt, R.G. Holloway, J.R. Curtis. Palliative care: a core competency for stroke neurologists. *Stroke*, 2015; 46(9): 2714–9.

10. B.R. Ferrell, M.L. Twaddle, A. Melnick, et al. National consensus project clinical practice guidelines for quality palliative care guidelines, 4th edition. *Journal of Palliative Medicine*, 2018; 21(12): 1684–9.

11. *America's care of serious illness: a state-by-state report card on access to palliative care in our nation's hospitals.* New York: Center to Advance Palliative Care and the National Palliative Care Research Center; 2019.

12. R. Aslakson, J. Cheng, D. Vollenweider, D. Galusca, T.J. Smith, P.J. Pronovost. Evidence-based palliative care in the intensive care unit: a systematic review of interventions. *Journal of Palliative Medicine*, 2014; 17(2): 219–35.

13. J.E. Nelson, R. Bassett, R.D. Boss, et al. Models for structuring a clinical initiative to enhance palliative care in the intensive care unit: a report from the IPAL-ICU Project (Improving Palliative Care in the ICU). *Critical Care Medicine*, 2010; 38(9): 1765–72.

14. S.A. Norton, L.A. Hogan, R.G. Holloway, et al. Proactive palliative care in the medical intensive care unit: effects on length of stay for selected high-risk patients. *Critical Care Medicine*, 2007; 35(6): 1530–5.

15. R.J. Zalenski, S.S. Jones, C. Courage, et al. Impact of palliative care screening and consultation in the ICU: a multihospital quality improvement project. *Journal of Pain and Symptom Management*, 2017; 53(1): 5–12.e3.

16. M.L. Campbell, J.A. Guzman. A proactive approach to improve end-of-life care in a medical intensive care unit for patients with terminal dementia. *Critical Care Medicine*, 2004; 32(9): 1839.

17. A.C. Mosenthal, P.A. Murphy, L.K. Barker, et al. Livingston. Changing the culture around end-of-life care in the trauma intensive care unit. *Journal of Trauma*, 2008; 64(6): 1587–93.

18. S. Lamba, P. Murphy, S. McVicker, et al. Changing end-of-life care practice for liver transplant service patients: structured palliative care intervention in the surgical intensive care unit. *Journal of Pain and Symptom Management*, 2012; 44(4): 508–19.

19. R.S. Morrison, J.D. Penrod, J.B. Cassel, et al. Cost savings associated with US hospital palliative care consultation programs. *Archives of Internal Medicine*, 2008; 168(16): 1783–90.

20. M. Kaufer, P. Murphy, K. Barker, et al. Family satisfaction following the death of a loved one in an inner city MICU. *American Journal of Hospice and Palliative Medicine*, 2008; 25(4): 318–25.

21. C.E. Cox, C.L. Lewis, L.C. Hanson, et al. Development and pilot testing of a decision aid for surrogates of patients with prolonged mechanical ventilation. *Critical Care Medicine*, 2012; 40(8): 2327–34.

22. E. Azoulay, F. Pochard, S. Chevret, et al. Impact of a family information leaflet on effectiveness of information provided to family members of intensive care unit patients: a multicenter, prospective, randomized, controlled trial. *Am J Respir Critical Care Medicine*, 2002; 165(4): 438–42.

23. J.P. Burns, M.M. Mello, D.M. Studdert, et al. Results of a clinical trial on care improvement for the critically ill. *Critical Care Medicine*, 2003; 31(8): 2107–17.

24. D.B. White, S.M. Cua, R. Walk, et al. Nurse-led intervention to improve surrogate decision making for patients with advanced critical illness. *American Journal of Critical Care*, 2012; 21(6): 396–409.

25. D.B. White, D.C. Angus, A-M. et al. A Randomized trial of a family-support intervention in intensive care units. *New England Journal of Medicine*, 2018; 378 (25): 2365–75.

26. J.R. Curtis, P.D. Treece, E.L. Nielsen, et al. Randomized trial of communication facilitators to reduce family distress and intensity of end-of-life care. *American Journal of Respiratory and Critical Care Medicine*, 2015; 193(2): 154–62.

27. A. Lautrette, D. Michael, M. Bruno, et al. A communication strategy and brochure for relatives of patients dying in the ICU. *New England Journal of Medicine*, 2007; 356: 469–78.

28. C.M. Lilly, D.L. De Meo, L.A. Sonna, et al. An intensive communication intervention for the critically ill. *American Journal of Medicine* 2000; 109(6): 469–75.

29. C. Lilly, L. Sonna, K. Haley, et al. Intensive communication: four-year follow-up from a clinical practice study. *Critical Care Medicine*, 2003; 31(5 Suppl): S394–9.

30. T.E. Quill, A.P. Abernethy. Generalist plus specialist palliative care – creating a more sustainable model. *New England Journal of Medicine*, 2013; 368: 1173–5.

31. L. Sihra, M. Harris, C. O'Reardon. Using the improving palliative care in the intensive care unit (IPAL-ICU) project to promote palliative care consultation. *Journal of Pain and Symptom Management*, 2011; 42(5): 672–5.

32. C.T. Bradley, K.J. Brasel. Developing guidelines that identify patients who would benefit from palliative care services in the surgical intensive care unit. *Critical Care Medicine*, 2009; 37(3): 946.

33. M.T. Williams, E. Zimmerman, M. Barry, et al. A retrospective review of patients with acute stroke with and without palliative care consultations. *American Journal of Hospice and Palliative Care*, 2019; 36(1): 60–4.

34. T. Singh, S.R. Peters, D.L. Tirschwell, et al. Palliative care for hospitalized patients with stroke. *Stroke*, 2017; 48(9): 2534–40.

35. C. Creutzfeldt, R. Engelberg, L. Healey, et al. Palliative care needs in the neuro-ICU. *Critical Care Medicine*, 2015; 43(8): 1677–84.

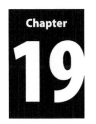

Measuring and Evaluating Shared Decision-Making in the Intensive Care Unit

Alison E. Turnbull and
Jacqueline M. Kruser

Shared experiences are inherently challenging to measure and evaluate, and shared decision-making (SDM) in the context of critical illness is no exception. The shared nature of a decision is an abstract idea, or latent construct. Declaring a specific decision to have been shared requires knowing how multiple parties viewed their roles in this complex process. As a result, there are few validated instruments that have been successfully used to measure SDM in the intensive care unit (ICU) setting.

Nevertheless, policymakers generally agree that SDM is fundamental to high-quality ICU care and often seek to quantify or evaluate its occurrence. Most approaches to evaluating SDM assess one of three things: (1) system-level infrastructure and policy hypothesized to impact SDM, (2) steps or features of the decision-making process at the level of individual decisions for individual patients, or (3) patient-, clinician-, and family-reported outcomes that the SDM process is hypothesized to affect (Figure 19.1). Selecting a method depends on careful consideration of the question you seek to answer.

19.1 Infrastructure and Policy

The underlying structure of a health-care system can impact patient care in important ways. Organizational priorities, ICU-specific culture, and the physical layout and practical resources of ICUs can influence the frequency and quality of SDM. And although unit- and hospital-level structural measures alone do not guarantee that SDM occurs, they can provide an indirect indication of the value placed on SDM within an institution when patient-level data collection is prohibitively expensive or labor intensive.

Physical infrastructure measures may involve assessing the availability of structural resources that promote family and proxy decision maker presence in the ICU, as well as resources that facilitate patient participation in SDM. Examples of physical infrastructure recommended to facilitate SDM include a dedicated and appropriately furnished room for meetings between clinicians and family members, and individual patient rooms that include comfortable

INFRASTRUCTURE AND POLICY MEASURES

Unit- and hospital-level measures of resources, policies, and procedures that support shared decision making.

DECISION-MAKING PROCESS MEASURES

Decision-level measures that evaluate whether a specific encounter met a set of criteria for shared decision making.

PATIENT, FAMILY, AND CLINICIAN OUTCOME MEASURES

Patient, family, and clincian-level measures of the effects of the decision or decision-making process on stakeholders.

Figure 19.1 Structure, process, and outcomes: Three tiers of SDM measures.

spaces and facilities for visitors (i.e., showers) so that patient proxies are more likely to be available for discussions. Other unit-level measures of the resources that promote patient involvement in SDM include availability of speaking valves for ventilated patients, other resources to facilitate speech during invasive mechanical ventilation (i.e., expertise with deflated cuff speech), and communication support devices such as communication boards.[1–3]

Infrastructure related to the electronic medical record (EMR) can also provide insights into the system-level facilitation of SDM. Elements of EMR design that support SDM include dedicated, easily accessible, and editable features that (1) store legal documents such as advance directives and portable medical orders related to life-sustaining treatments (i.e., physician orders for life-sustaining treatment forms), (2) store the identity and contact information of patient health-care proxies, and (3) document the content and outcomes of discussions that take place between clinicians, patients, their proxies, and other friends and family members.

The interprofessional staffing of ICUs varies greatly and can impact both the timing and quality of SDM. Interpreters, social workers, palliative care consultants, chaplains, and clinical ethics consultants often play important roles in SDM. However, not all hospitals and ICUs have each of these professionals on staff, and their hours may be limited to weekday business hours.

Finally, policies written and implemented at the ICU, hospital, and institutional levels can explicitly address SDM, or indirectly signal how patients and families are viewed. For example, some institutions have decision-making protocols for high-risk procedures such as extracorporeal life support or ventricular assist devices. Policies and protocols that support SDM could require family meetings, palliative care consultation, ethics consultation, or signed agreements about the administration and duration of therapies. An investigator using this approach to understanding attitudes toward SDM in a health system might survey ICUs about unit-level policies regarding visiting hours, the number of family members who can be in a patient's room, family presence during rounds, and family presence during invasive procedures or cardiopulmonary resuscitation. The presence of SDM curriculum for medical trainees and the educational resources dedicated to ensuring physicians are skilled at engaging with proxies when making decisions also signal the cultural importance of SDM within teaching institutions.

19.2 The Decision-Making Process

Before assessing what roles two parties played in the process of making a decision about healthcare, investigators must first determine what needs to be decided and whether the decision warrants SDM. Most decisions made in an ICU are appropriately not made in collaboration with patients or their families. These include medical decisions like what ventilator settings to apply, what dose of antibiotics or analgesics to give, and what diagnostic test to order. According to a 2016 joint policy statement from The American College of Critical Care Medicine and the American Thoracic Society, "clinicians should engage in a SDM process to define overall goals of care and when making major treatment decisions that may be affected by personal values, goals, and preferences."[4] Although there is general consensus that decisions about code status, as well as withholding and withdrawing life support fit these criteria, deciding what other interventions constitute preference-sensitive decisions is not always so straightforward. Investigators may choose to focus on a single procedure that clearly requires the consideration of a patient's goals and limits, such as a tracheostomy for patients with prolonged mechanical ventilation and a poor prognosis. Alternatively, a modified Delphi process can help to achieve consensus among stakeholders about a panel of interventions requiring SDM.[5]

An investigator's next challenge is identifying each potential opportunity for SDM about the decision of interest. In a prospective study, this means anticipating when the clinical team will engage the patient or their surrogate. A member of the research team may need to round or coordinate closely with the clinical team throughout the day so they are prepared to record or observe family meetings or similar interactions. In a retrospective study, investigators must rely on the EMR for evidence of a SDM process. However, caution is warranted when using the EMR to identify instances of SDM because documentation may be incomplete or inconsistent.

Clinicians' narrative accounts of decision-making can usually be found within EMR progress notes. Progress notes may include clinician rationales, longitudinal accounts of events, and narrative comments that lend depth to understanding a patient's hospital stay (Table 19.1). Some EMRs also have unique note types for documenting events relevant to SDM, such as family meetings. These textual data can be analyzed using qualitative methods[6] or natural language processing.[7] However, EMR documentation is unlikely to describe all relevant communication, and typically only provides a clinician's perspective.

Fields within an EMR, distinct from the narrative progress notes, can indicate whether the patient has decision-making capacity, the patient's legal healthcare proxy (or the steps taken to declare a patient unbefriended), contact information for that legal proxy, and copies of legal documents pertaining to decision-making about the patient's care such as advance directives and physician orders for life-sustaining treatment forms.

There are dozens of instruments designed to evaluate the SDM process from the perspective of patients or proxies, providers, and observers.[8] However, these instruments vary in quality and most have not been validated in the ICU setting. Herein, we highlight select instruments that have been most widely used or are likely to be responsive and feasible in the ICU setting and are immune to floor and ceiling effects. Investigators who are interested in whether patients or proxies possess the requisite knowledge to make an informed decision may choose to supplement these process measures with standardized questionnaires about the specific risks and benefits of the decision of interest.

Measurement instruments which ask ICU patient surrogates to report on their experience via structured questionnaires are called proxy-reported experience measures (PREMS). When using PREMS to evaluate the SDM process, a few caveats should be kept in mind. The first is that proxies prefer varying levels of control and involvement in preference-sensitive decisions. The same proxy may eschew involvement in low-stakes decisions but prefer total control of value-laden decisions about a patient's death.[9] Second, when asked if they shared in the decision-making process, people tend to interpret the question as asking if they are satisfied with their

Table 19.1. Stakeholders' roles in the evaluation of SDM in the ICU

Stakeholder	Data source	Examples and instruments	Considerations
Patients	Patient-reported experience measures	QOC	Not feasible for patients who are unconscious, delirious, or lack capacity
	Patient-reported outcome measures	Survival, place of residence	Only available for ICU survivors and not a direct measure of SDM
Proxy decision makers, or family members	PREMS	QOC, Decisional Conflict Scale, collaboRATE, PPPC, FS-ICU	Scales developed for the outpatient setting and may require modification for ICU
	Proxy-reported knowledge measures	Proxy understanding of risks and benefits of specific treatment options	Knowledge is sensitive to the timing of data collection and not a direct measure of SDM.
	Proxy-reported outcome measures	Decisional Regret, HADS, IES-R	Proxy psychological outcomes affected by complex influences beyond SDM
Clinicians	Clinician-reported experience	Qualitative analysis and natural language processing of narrative notes in EMR	Medical record is incomplete record of communication and SDM process
	Clinician evaluations of care	Clinician evaluations of the concordance between patient goals and care received	Methodologies are nascent and untested
	Clinician-reported outcomes	Moral Distress Scale-Revised Maslach Burnout Inventory	Exploratory only; relationship of SDM has not been clearly established
Researchers and other external observers	Infrastructure and policy evaluation	EMR design, availability of consultants to facilitate SDM, visitation policies	Structural support does not guarantee that SDM occurs for individual patients
	Discrete process and outcome measures derived from EMR	Family meeting occurrence and timing, code status, discharge disposition	EMR documentation may be inconsistent and may not reflect actual events

Table 19.1. (cont.)

Stakeholder	Data source	Examples and instruments	Considerations
	Audio or video-recorded interactions between proxies and clinicians	OPTION(5) Scale, Patient-Centeredness of Care Scale	External observers may improve measure objectivity but can be resource -intensive

Abbreviations: FS-ICU, Family Satisfaction with the ICU Survey; HADS, Hospital Anxiety and Depression Scale; IES-R, Impact of Event Scale-Revised; PPPC, Patient-Perception of Patient-Centeredness; PREMS, proxy-reported experience measures; QOC, Quality of Communication Questionnaire

provider or their care,[10] which is often associated with a provider's age, accent, gender, and race. Therefore, PREMS should be interpreted cautiously. Finally, enrolling a representative sample of ICU proxies can be challenging. Patients near death and those from wealthy neighborhoods are most likely to have a family member available at the bedside.[11] Proxies whose loved ones receive palliative care have also historically been more willing to participate in research,[12] which may generate a cohort with disproportionately high exposure to SDM.

Despite these obstacles, PREMS are routinely used in the ICU. The six-item general communication skills score within the Quality of Communication Questionnaire[13] has been used extensively and asks whether doctors spoke understandably, made eye contact, listened, answered questions, paid attention, and seemed to care about the patient. The Decisional Conflict Scale captures how emotionally distressed a proxy feels about a specific decision with scores ranging from 0 to 100.[14,15] The Patient Perception of Patient-Centeredness (PPPC) is a 14-item scale originally developed for use in the outpatient setting.[16] However, modified versions of the PPPC have been used to evaluate communication interventions in the ICU setting,[17] and PPPC scores are associated with satisfaction with the information provided by clinicians.[18] Finally, the three-item collaboRATE scale[19] is designed for evaluating the level of SDM in encounters that included multiple decisions. It includes a version for patient proxies and is available under a Creative Commons license.

Observer measures of SDM use trained assessors, who are often researchers, to assess audio- or video-recorded encounters. Recording ICU encounters and training assessors is labor intensive, time consuming, and requires informed consent from all participants. However, it also allows for a detailed evaluation of clinician behavior, including core aspects of SDM, such as highlighting the existence of a choice, eliciting patient preferences, and explaining options. One approach developed for evaluating SDM in the outpatient setting[20] and successfully adapted for research in the ICU setting[21] involves a third party assessing whether physicians performed 10 behaviors central to SDM. These actions include describing treatment alternatives, discussing uncertainty, and assessing understanding. The OPTION(5) measure,[22] which is applicable to a wide variety of clinical circumstances, is similar and was designed to minimize assessor burden. Although not specifically designed to assess SDM, the Patient-Centeredness of Care Scale[16,23] also involves experts coding how doctors respond to patient or family statements during an observed or recorded encounter.

Combining data from multiple sources may minimize the limitations inherent in each source. For example, the Dyadic OPTION instrument collects data from a patient or proxy–clinician dyad and compares how each party perceived elements of SDM during an encounter.[24] Comparing the patient preferences reported by ICU proxies to notes and orders in the medical record can also provide an indirect assessment of proxy involvement in decisions about care.[25] Comparing PREMS with the medical record, or observer methods performed by clinical researchers, can create a more complete picture of how all parties in the room perceived a decision-making event.

19.3 Outcomes of SDM

Supporting critically ill patients and their loved ones who wish to make informed choices about their medical care is arguably a worthwhile and ethical goal regardless of whether it impacts the care received. However, sustained changes in medical practice are rarely the result of ethics-based, deontological motivation.[26] Even an intervention that increases patient or family understanding, satisfaction, and engagement in decision-making while decreasing decisional conflict and regret is unlikely to be consistently implemented if it requires clinician time and does not substantially improve outcomes. Therefore, any evaluation of an intervention designed to promote or improve SDM in the ICU setting should consider assessing outcomes valued by a range of stakeholders.

19.4 Patient Outcomes

Evaluations focused on SDM about a specific intervention, treatment, or procedure, should strive to estimate rates of various outcomes by collecting data on both the number of patients for whom a decision was required (denominator), and the number of patients with each possible outcome of the SDM process (numerator). Investigators should also consider evaluating change in the timing of decisions (i.e., the ICU day of SDM events); however, caution is needed when evaluating the rate of specific interventions. In most cases, there is no ideal intervention rate toward which a care team should aim.

Rather, interventions should be performed because they are expected to help an individual patient reach a valued and achievable goal.[27] To truly understand whether care is improving an evaluation should strive to assess the incidence of goal-concordant care. Unfortunately, methodologies for assessing the goal-concordance of specific interventions[27,28] and a patient's overall care[29] are nascent and not well-validated.

The effect of SDM interventions on short- and long-term survival should also be assessed. ICU patients who are unlikely to live more than a few months and are supported to participate in SDM may prefer to stop treatment and die in the hospital. As a result, an SDM intervention may affect the rate of survival to hospital discharge, without changing the 3- to 6-month mortality rate. Other important outcomes to consider include length of stay and hospital discharge disposition, which have been responsive to ICU communication interventions in prior studies.[30] Finally, semistructured interviews with ICU survivors[31] and patient-reported outcomes including satisfaction and quality of life after discharge can improve our understanding of SDM, but they are subject to survival bias.

19.5 Proxy Outcomes

The majority of ICU patients lack capacity for decision-making at some point during their ICU stay,[32] so SDM interventions in the ICU setting are typically designed for proxy decision-makers. The Decision Regret Scale[33] was designed to measure regret about healthcare decisions in patients, and a modified version can be administered to proxies of critically ill adults; users should recognize, however, that levels of regret among ICU proxies, including about end-of-life decisions, are generally very low.[34] Commonly assessed SDM outcomes are proxies' symptoms of depression and post-traumatic stress. There are multiple screening tools available for assessing these potential mental health sequelae of decision-making responsibility in the ICU, such as the Hospital Anxiety and Depression Scale[35] and the Impact of Event Scale – Revised.[36] However, proxy mental health symptoms are affected by multiple, complex influences beyond SDM and previously studied ICU interventions to improve these symptoms have generally failed to demonstrate an effect. Proxies with post-traumatic stress symptoms may also avoid completing questionnaires that ask them to recall a traumatic experience, creating the potential for differential loss to follow-up.

19.6 Clinician and Institutional Outcomes

Sharing requires compromise. ICU clinicians who engage in SDM often need to negotiate and compromise about care plans with family members experiencing strong emotions. This work is difficult, and evaluations of SDM should consider its potential impact on clinicians. Clinician outcome measures to consider include burnout,[37] moral distress,[38] job satisfaction, and staff turnover. Evaluations of interventions to foster or improve SDM should also consider collecting data on outcomes of importance to institutional administrators including the incidence of calls to a hospital's patient relations service, requests for assistance from hospital security, requests for facilitation or mediation by chaplains, palliative care, clinical ethics, or risk management/legal counsel services.

Acknowledgments

The authors thank Ian M. Oppenheim, MD, and Emma M. Lee for their input and proofreading.

References

1. D.C. Tippett, A.A. Siebens. Using ventilators for speaking and swallowing. *Dysphagia*, 1991; 6(2):94–9.

2. J.D. Hoit, R.B. Banzett, H.L. Lohmeier, et al. Clinical ventilator adjustments that improve speech. *Chest*, 2003; 124(4): 1512–21.

3. J.R. Bach, A.S. Alba. Tracheostomy ventilation. A study of efficacy with deflated cuffs and cuffless tubes. *Chest*, 1990; 97(3): 679–83.

4. A.A. Kon, J.E. Davidson, W. Morrison, et al. Shared decision making in ICUs: an American College of Critical Care Medicine and American Thoracic Society Policy Statement. *Critical Care Medicine*, 2016; 44(1): 188–201.

5. A.E. Turnbull, S.K. Sahetya, D.M. Needham. Aligning critical care interventions with patient goals: a modified Delphi study. *Heart & Lung*, 2016; 45(6): 517–24.

6. S.P.Y. Wong, E.K. Vig, J.S. Taylor, et al. Timing of initiation of maintenance dialysis: a qualitative analysis of the electronic medical records of a national cohort of patients from the Department of Veterans Affairs. *JAMA Internal Medicine*, 2016; 176(2): 228–35.

7. G.E. Weissman, R.A. Hubbard, L.H. Ungar, et al. Inclusion of unstructured clinical text improves early prediction of death or prolonged ICU stay. *Critical Care Medicine*, 2018; 46(7): 1125–32.

8. F.R. Gärtner, H. Bomhof-Roordink, I.P. Smith, et al. The quality of instruments to assess the process of shared decision making: a systematic review. *PLoS ONE*, 2018; 13(2): e0191747.

9. S.K. Johnson, C.A. Bautista, S.Y. Hong, et al. An empirical study of surrogates' preferred level of control over value-laden life support decisions in intensive care units. *American Journal of Respiratory and Critical Care Medicine*, 2011; 183(7): 915–21.

10. V. Entwistle, M. Prior, Z.C. Skea, et al. Involvement in treatment decision-making: its meaning to people with diabetes and implications for conceptualisation. *Social Science & Medicine*, 2008; 66(2): 362–75.

11. A.E. Turnbull, M.D. Hashem, A. Rabiee, et al. Evaluation of a strategy for enrolling the families of critically ill patients in research using limited human resources. *PLoS ONE*, 2017; 12(5): e0177741.

12. E.K. Kross, R.A. Engelberg, S.E. Shannon, et al. Potential for response bias in family surveys about end-of-life care in the ICU. *Chest*, 2009; 136(6): 1496–502.

13. R. Engelberg, L. Downey, J.R. Curtis. Psychometric characteristics of a quality of communication questionnaire assessing communication about end-of-life care. *Journal of Palliative Medicine*, 2006; 9(5): 1086–98.

14. A.M. O'Connor. Validation of a decisional conflict scale. *Medical Decision Making*, 1995; 15(1): 25–30.

15. J. Chiarchiaro, P. Buddadhumaruk, R.M. Arnold, et al. Prior advance care planning is associated with less decisional conflict among surrogates for critically ill patients. *Annals of the American Thoracic Society*, 2015; 12(10): 1528–33.

16. M. Stewart, J.B. Brown, A. Donner, et al. The impact of patient-centered care on outcomes. *Journal of Family Practice*, 2000; 49(9): 796–804.

17. D.B. White, D.C. Angus, A.M. Shields, et al. A randomized trial of a family-support intervention in intensive care units. *New England Journal of Medicine*, 2018; 378(25): 2365–75.

18. J.B. Mallinger, J.J. Griggs, C.G. Shields. Patient-centered care and breast cancer survivors' satisfaction with information. *Patient Education and Counseling*, 2005; 57 (3): 342–9.

19. P.J. Barr, R. Thompson, T. Walsh, et al. The psychometric properties of CollaboRATE: a fast and frugal patient-reported measure of the shared decision-making process. *Journal of Medical Internet Research*, 2014; 16(1): e2.

20. C.H.B. Iii, K.A. Edwards, N.M. Hasenberg, et al. Informed decision making in outpatient practice: time to get back to basics. *JAMA* 1999; 282(24): 2313–20.

21. D.B. White, C.H. Braddock, S. Bereknyei, et al. Toward shared decision making at the end of life in intensive care units: opportunities for improvement. *Archives of Internal Medicine*, 2007; 167(5): 461–7.

22. P.J. Barr, A.J. O'Malley, M. Tsulukidze, et al. The psychometric properties of Observer OPTION(5), an observer measure of shared decision making. *Patient Education and Counseling*, 2015; 98(8): 970–6.

23. R.J. Henbest, M.A. Stewart. Patient-centredness in the consultation. 1: a method for measurement. *Family Practice*, 1989; 6(4): 249–53.

24. E. Melbourne, S. Roberts, M-A. Durand, et al. Dyadic OPTION: measuring perceptions of shared decision-making in practice. *Patient Education and Counseling*, 2011; 83(1): 55–7.

25. A.E. Turnbull, C.M. Chessare, R.K. Coffin, et al. More than one in three proxies do not know their loved one's current code status: an observational study in a Maryland ICU. *PLoS ONE*, 2019; 14(1): e0211531.

26. G. Elwyn, D.L. Frosch, S. Kobrin. Implementing shared decision-making: consider all the consequences. *Implementation Science*, 2016; 11(1): 114.

27. A.E. Turnbull, C.S. Hartog. Goal-concordant care in the ICU: A conceptual framework for future research. *Intensive Care Medicine*, 2017; 43(12): 1847–9.

28. A.E. Turnbull, S.K. Sahetya, E. Colantuoni, et al. Inter-rater agreement of intensivists evaluating the goal concordance of preference-sensitive ICU interventions. *Journal of Pain and Symptom Management*, 2018; 56(3): 406–13.

29. S.D. Halpern. Goal-concordant care – Searching for the Holy Grail. *New England Journal of Medicine*, 2019; 381(17): 1603–6.

30. A.E. Turnbull, G.T. Bosslet, E.K. Kross. Aligning use of intensive care with patient values in the USA: past, present, and future. *Lancet Respiratory Medicine*, 2019; 7(7): 626–38.

31. D.J. Lamas, R.L. Owens, R.N. Nace, et al. Opening the door: the experience of chronic critical illness in a long-term acute care hospital. *Critical Care Medicine*, 2017; 45(4): e357–62.

32. A.M. Torke, G.A. Sachs, P.R. Helft, et al. Scope and outcomes of surrogate decision making among hospitalized older adults. *JAMA Internal Medicine*, 2014; 174(3): 370–7.

33. J.C. Brehaut, A.M. O'Connor, T.J. Wood, et al. Validation of a decision regret scale. *Medical Decision Making*, 2003; 23(4): 281–92.

34. J.J. Miller, P. Morris, D.C. Files, et al. Decision conflict and regret among surrogate decision makers in the medical intensive care unit. *Journal of Critical Care*, 2016; 32: 79–84.

35. A.S. Zigmond, R.P. Snaith. The hospital anxiety and depression scale. *Acta Psychiatrica Scandinavica*, 1983; 67(6): 361–70.

36. J.G. Beck, D.M. Grant, J.P. Read, et al. The impact of event scale-revised: psychometric properties in a sample of motor vehicle accident survivors. *Journal of Anxiety Disorders*, 2008; 22(2): 187–98.

37. S.M. Pastores, V. Kvetan, C.M. Coopersmith, et al. Workforce, workload, and burnout among intensivists and advanced practice providers: a narrative review. *Critical Care Medicine*, 2019; 47(4): 550–7.

38. K.W. Altaker, J. Howie-Esquivel, J.K. Cataldo. Relationships among palliative care, ethical climate, empowerment, and moral distress in intensive care unit nurses. *American Journal of Critical Care*, 2018; 27(4): 295–302.

Chapter 20

Brain Death Discussions

Elizabeth Carroll and Ariane Lewis

In 1959, shortly after the invention of positive pressure ventilation, Pierre Mollaret and Maurice Goulon published the first description of what would eventually be referred to as "brain death" in their manuscript "Le Coma Depassé."[1,2] Nearly a decade later, a committee commissioned by Harvard Medical School expanded on Mollaret and Goulon's work and described their acceptance of the use of neurologic criteria to declare death when a person is unreceptive and unresponsive, does not move or breathe, has absent reflexes, and has an isoelectric electroencephalogram.[2,3] In the ensuing 50 years, the use of neurologic criteria to declare death has become medically and legally accepted as death throughout much of the world.[4,5]

Despite this, many people do not understand the concept of brain death, and among those who understand it, some object to it.[6-8] This confusion can largely be attributed to the fact that most knowledge the public has about brain death comes from television, movies, and media, all of which can be misleading, at best, or grossly inaccurate, at worst.[9-11] There are also varying religious perspectives on brain death, some of which prompt objections to the use of neurologic criteria to declare death.[12-18] These factors can make communication about brain death challenging.

Here, as a final Chapter for this book that covers a wide variety of potentially challenging discussions with families, we tackle one of the most difficult. We provide data on how well providers communicate about brain death, review strategies to discuss brain death, address objections to brain death, then close by briefly discussing organ donation after brain death. Of note, although it is beyond the scope of this Chapter, we remind the reader that, when thinking about brain death, it is imperative that providers (1) review the guidelines for brain death determination, (2) consider pitfalls in brain death determination, including brain death mimics, and (3) familiarize themselves with local laws about brain death.

20.1 Data on the Effectiveness of Communication About Brain Death

The subject of brain death is arguably one of the most difficult topics for health-care providers to discuss with a patient's family, given poor public understanding of the topic and lack of guidance for healthcare providers on how to approach these discussions.[10] In a review of brain death protocols from around the world, Lewis et al. discovered that only 36% of protocols addressed the need to communicate with a patient's family prior to declaration of brain death and only 12% noted the importance of communicating with a patient's family prior to discontinuation of organ support.[19]

A discussion of the ideal ways to communicate about brain death is important because studies have shown that health-care providers sometimes fail to adequately educate family members about this complicated topic.[20] In a study by the National Kidney Foundation, nearly one-third of donor family members of brain dead patients wished they were told more information about brain death.[21] Savaria et al found that 15% of donor family members did not have a clear understanding of brain death.[22] In interviews of the immediate next of kin of 164 medically suitable organ donor candidates, 39% of respondents said brain death was not explained to them and 20% did not understand that brain death is irreversible.[21]

20.2 Communicating About Brain Death

The fact that some families are inadequately educated about brain death is reflective of the fact that discussing brain death with a person's family can be an incredibly difficult task for health-care providers. Who should discuss brain death, what should be said, when should it be said, where should it be said, and how should the conversation be structured?[17] We dissect the answers to these questions herein (Tables 20.1 and 20.2).

20.2.1 Who Should Be Involved in Discussions About Brain Death?

Providers should ensure that all members of the care team (clinicians, nurses, therapists, social workers, case managers, and patient care technicians) have a proper understanding of brain death and are aware of the potential for a brain death evaluation so that families are provided with consistent information. Providers who have a close therapeutic relationship with the family should introduce brain death in conjunction with consultants who are involved in brain death determination. Palliative care consultation should be considered, because they can offer an additional support system for families both during hospitalization and after discharge.

Table 20.1. Recommendations on how to talk to families about brain death

Review imaging of the patient's brain and explain what is abnormal

Allow families to observe your examination, explain your findings, and describe how they compare to normal findings

Begin education about the possibility of progression to brain death early when it is clear there has been a devastating neurologic injury

Ensure that the entire medical team understands the implications of the brain death examination so that information given to the family is consistent

Involve ethics, palliative care, social work, psychology, hospital chaplaincy, and/or a spiritual guide early in the admission

Provide frequent education and reeducation about brain death including details on the examination, the possibility of spinal reflexes, the legal implications of declaration of brain death, and the discontinuation of organ support after declaration of brain death

Communicate candidly and patiently

Establish a bond of trust with the family

Express sadness and empathize with the family's disbelief and grief

Use consistent terminology and layman's terms

Allow family to gather and perform religious rituals prior to the confirmatory examination

After declaration, use the term "death" not "brain death" to avoid being unclear

20.2.2 What Should Providers Tell Families About Brain Death?

Providers should begin discussions about brain death by informing a person's family that they suffered a catastrophic brain injury. They should disclose the etiology for this injury and demonstrate the extent of the injury on brain imaging. Additionally, they should both explain and demonstrate the neurologic examination before talking about brain death.

After establishing that an injury is severe and irreversible, providers should tell families that there are two types of death that are legally equivalent: (1) cardiopulmonary (traditional) death, which occurs when the heart and lungs stop working, and (2) brain death, which occurs when the entire brain stops working. They should further explain that when a person is brain dead, their heart and lungs only continue to function with the support of machines. Providers should then review their concerns that, in this case, the brain injury may be severe enough to cause brain death, but that a formal, thorough evaluation is necessary to meticulously assess for any signs of brain function.

Next, providers should describe the steps of the determination. They should begin by reviewing the prerequisites and the clinical examination in detail. It should be explained that any sign of brain activity during the

Table 20.2. Recommendations on things to say during discussions about brain death

"Brain death represents a devastating and irreversible neurologic injury incompatible with return of consciousness."

"I truly wish recovery were possible."

"This situation is terrible and I know that it happened very suddenly, which makes it even more stressful."

"We will do all we can, but in some cases, even when we do everything, a person dies."

"We need to ask – 'Who was this person before the accident?' Then explain, 'Based on our neurologic exam and tests, we have found that this person's brain has no function, and therefore, they have died. We can support their organs with these machines and medicines, but they have died. They will not wake up. The person you knew is gone.'"

"The only good thing here is that they are not experiencing any pain or discomfort. They are not suffering."

"The assessment is very detailed, so we can carefully evaluate for any evidence of brain activity. If there is any activity at all, that means they are still alive, but if there is no activity, that means they are dead."

"The point of the apnea test is to test the lowest portion of the brain. This part of the brain should trigger the lungs to breathe as carbon dioxide rises in the body. If this does not happen, it means that even the base of the brain is not working at all."

"Even though the brain is not working, there can sometimes still be reflexive movements due to activity from the spinal cord, the nerves, or the muscles. Although these are connected to the brain, and usually receive messages from the brain, they can send messages, sometimes, even when the brain isn't working. Movements that are coming from the brain are different from movements being triggered by the spinal cord, nerves, or muscles."

assessment indicates that a person is alive, but if there is no sign of brain activity during a clinical examination, the next step would be to perform apnea testing. When describing apnea testing, it is important for providers to reiterate that if a person takes a single breath, testing is aborted, because this demonstrates life, and if a person shows any signs of instability during the assessment, the ventilator is reconnected. Providers must explain that, during this period, the carbon dioxide in a person's body increases, and that if the base of the brain is working, this should trigger them to breathe. Families should be prepared for the potential for spinal reflexes and should be told that even when the brain is not working, the spine, muscles, and nerves can still show some activity. Additionally, providers should address the known or potential need for ancillary testing. Finally, providers should explain that if the clinical examination, apnea test, and ancillary test (if performed) reveal no signs of brain function, death will be declared, and that this will be the legal equivalence to cessation of the heart and lungs. Providers should disclose that, if a person is found to be brain dead, organ support will be discontinued.

Providers should invite families to observe brain death determination, as a recent randomized controlled trial suggested that this may improve understanding of brain death.[1,23] Importantly, this study demonstrated there was no apparent adverse effect of observing the determination on the psychological well-being of families. Providers should clearly explain the assessment and their findings during the assessment, if families are present, or after the assessment, if they are not.

20.2.3 When Should Providers Discuss Brain Death?

We recommend introducing the concept of brain death soon after it is evident that a person has suffered a catastrophic brain injury, if it is anticipated that they may progress to brain death. Although it may seem uncomfortable to discuss brain death shortly after meeting a family, it is best to prepare them and not delay the discussion. A lack of preparedness is associated with worse outcomes for families.[24] It is helpful to provide families with a general timeline of when the team plans to perform the neurologic exam, apnea testing, and ancillary testing (if applicable), so they can set their expectations accordingly and coordinate arrangements for other family members or religious advisors to be present. Within reason, providers should be somewhat flexible when discussing this timeline; this gives families an opportunity to accept the situation and allows additional family members to come to the hospital before the brain death determination.

Although we discuss this further, it is worth noting that we strongly recommend against introducing the concept of organ donation during early discussions about brain death. It is best to delay discussion of organ donation until a designated organ procurement representative is present to discuss donation.

20.2.4 Where Should Discussions About Brain Death Take Place?

Providers should ask families where they prefer to discuss prognosis. Some families may wish to stay at the bedside, whereas others may prefer to meet in a private conference room. Please refer to Chapter 4, "Communication Skills for Critical Care Family Meetings" for additional details regarding family meeting organization.

20.2.5 How Should Discussions About Brain Death Be Structured?

It is imperative that providers be empathetic and culturally sensitive when discussing brain death and avoid the use of medical jargon.

There is an abundance of literature describing effective communication techniques when delivering bad news, as discussed throughout this text, all of which are applicable to discussions about brain death. Three commonly used techniques include (1) SPIKES (Setup (prepare the room), Perception (determine what is known), Invitation (ask if one can discuss the planned topic), Knowledge (give knowledge clearly and unequivocally), Emotions (address and emphasize), Summarize the plan); (2) NURSE (Name the problem or emotion, Understand the origin of the issue, Respect (both verbal and nonverbal), Support, Explore the feeling); and (3) Ask–Tell–Ask[25] (see Chapter 4, "Communication Skills for Critical Care Family Meetings.")

Trevick et al. recommend a seven-step approach to communication with relatives of persons who may become brain dead.[24] The goal of this approach is to allow for an open line of communication and provide information in a timely manner. First, they recommend that providers (1) begin communicating with a person's relatives early, (2) explain the severity and nature of the injury, and (3) indicate that prognosis is definitively poor. Second, as a patient deteriorates, they advise that providers discuss the possibility of loss of all brain function. Third, they encourage providers to review the events that led to admission, summarize events to date, and communicate likelihood of brain death. Fourth, they advise providers to explain that brain death indicates death of a person and that a person who is brain dead is legally dead, and recommend avoidance of unclear phrases like "passed away" or "moved on." Fifth, they suggest providers ensure a family has adequate time to digest this information. Sixth, they instruct providers to facilitate discussions about organ donation with an organ procurement team. Last, they advise that providers offer families the opportunity to contact the intensive care unit team or organ procurement team after death with or without organ donation, as confusion, questions, and doubts may arise in the weeks or, even, months after death.

20.2.6 Why Is Effective Communication Important?

It is imperative to communicate about brain death in an effective manner and ensure that families have a clear understanding of brain death. Having a poor understanding of brain death can put families at increased risk for developing complicated grief and cause them to perseverate on the events that led up to the death.[23,26] Ineffective communication can also lead to moral distress for health-care providers. Last, although the facilitation of organ donation is never the goal of brain death determination, it is important to note that ineffective communication can negatively impact potential organ donation.[23,26]

20.3 Addressing Objections to the Use of Neurologic Criteria to Declare Death

Although brain death is legally equivalent to cardiac death throughout much of the world, families sometimes challenge the use of neurologic criteria to declare death or request continuation of organ support after brain death.[17,18]

These objections can be made for a number of reasons, including religious beliefs that death does not occur until the heart stops, belief that the recovery of neurologic function is possible, a desire to wait until additional family members arrive, or concern that the acceptance of brain death means giving up. Objections can be managed in a number of different ways, such as performance of a determination/discontinuation of organ support over a family's objection, provision of assistance to facilitate transfer to another facility, continuation of organ support for a finite period of time, or continuation of organ support until cardiopulmonary arrest.

The key things providers need to keep in mind when addressing objections to the use of neurologic criteria to declare death are (1) collaboration between health-care providers, hospital administration, the ethics team, and the legal team is necessary, (2) preparation is key, and (3) although every situation is unique, consistency is important.

Unfortunately, the majority of hospital protocols about brain death do not describe how to handle objections to brain death or withdrawal of organ support after brain death.[27] We believe a plan to address objections should be incorporated into all hospital policies on brain death to standardize management within a given institution, because variability can be confusing for families and the health-care team.[28] Legal and administrative teams should be involved in formulating these guidelines in conjunction with clinical and ethics teams.

Providers should be aware that the American Academy of Neurology has recommendations on management of objections to brain death determination.[29] Notably, they (1) indicate that providers have both the "moral authority and professional responsibility, when lawful, to perform a brain death evaluation...after informing a patient's loved ones...without obligation to obtain informed consent" and (2) acknowledge that, both legally and ethically, autonomy is not absolute and does not necessitate that families have the right to demand unjustified medical treatment such as provision of prolonged organ support after brain death.

However, providers need to be aware of local laws about management of objections to brain death, because these can vary, and seek legal and administrative guidance when addressing objections.[30]

As discussed, providers can take many different actions when a family objects to the use of neurologic criteria to declare death. Although it may seem compassionate to continue organ support after brain death to allow families to come to terms with a person's death, the delay between brain death and cardiopulmonary arrest can be lengthy.[31,32] Continuing support for a protracted period in this setting can (1) promote confusion about a person's status and increase the risk for the family to develop complicated grief; (2) be stressful for health-care providers; and (3) divert resources, such as an intensive care unit bed, away from patients with the potential for recovery.[17,18,33]

20.4 Organ Donation After Brain Death

It is generally not the job of the providers involved in a person's medical care to address organ donation, given that this can suggest a conflict of interest and a family may perceive the purpose of brain death determination is to facilitate organ donation. Because of this, the discussion of organ donation should be left to the organ procurement team.[1] However, it is often the job of health-care providers to reach out to the organ procurement team and assist the team and family as needed. Of course, the health-care team should not treat a family any differently regardless of whether or not they agree to organ donation.[23] Notably, data suggest that bringing up the possibility of organ donation before a declaration of brain death is associated with greater donation authorization rates.[26]

Although the job of raising the possibility of organ donation with the patient's family is often left to the organ procurement organization, the health-care team should be prepared to take part in, and even lead such conversations, if family members raise the topic themselves. Providers should be aware that fear often surrounds the process of organ donation; families may voice concerns about disfigurement of the body or cost of the process.[26,34] It is important to provide reassurance and factual explanations about organ donation. It can also be helpful to mention the number of lives that donation can save. Providers should consistently encourage families to focus on patient wishes. Finally, it is imperative to encourage families to ask questions throughout the process.

20.5 Conclusion

Discussions about brain death require (1) expertise about brain death and the criteria for brain death determination, (2) empathy, (3) cultural sensitivity, (4) proficiency at communication and education about brain death, and (5) skills at answering questions about brain death and managing objections to brain death. Health-care providers involved in brain death determination should be trained in both the technical aspects of determination and the ideal methodology to facilitate conversations about brain death.[25,35]

References

1. T.S. Youn, D.M. Greer. Brain death and management of a potential organ donor in the intensive care unit. *Critical Care Clinics*, 2014; 30(4): 813–31.

2. P. Mollaret, M. Goulon. Le coma depasse. *Revue Neurologique*, 1959; 101: 3–15.

3. A definition of irreversible coma. Report of the Ad Hoc Committee of the Harvard Medical School to Examine the Definition of Brain Death. *JAMA*, 1968; 205(6): 337–40.

4. S. Wahlster, E. Wijdicks, P. Patel, et al. Brain death declaration: Practices and perceptions worldwide. *Neurology*. 2015; 84(18): 1870–9.

5. S.D. Shemie, L. Hornby, A. Baker, J. et al. International guideline development for the determination of death. *Intensive Care Medicine*, 2014; 40(6): 788–97.

6. A.F. Kocaay, S.U. Celik, T. Eker, et al. Brain death and organ donation: Knowledge, awareness, and attitudes of medical, law, divinity, nursing, and communication students. *Transplant Proceedings*, 2015; 47(5): 1244–8.

7. N. Wig, P. Gupta, S. Kailash. Awareness of brain death and organ transplantation among select Indian population. *Journal of the Association of Physicians of India*, 2003; 51: 455–8.

8. K.K. Bedi, A.R. Hakeem, R. Dave, et al. Survey of the knowledge, perception, and attitude of medical students at the University of Leeds toward organ donation and transplantation. *Transplant Proceedings*, 2015; 47(2): 247–60.

9. A. Lewis, J. Weaver, A. Caplan. Portrayal of brain death in film and television. *American Journal of Transplantation*, 2017; 17(3): 761–9.

10. A. Lewis, A.S. Lord, B.M. Czeisler, A. Caplan. Public education and misinformation on brain death in mainstream media. *Clinical Transplantation*, 2016; 30(9): 1082–9.

11. A. Daoust, E. Racine. Depictions of "brain death" in the media: Medical and ethical implications. *Journal of Medical Ethics*, 2014; 40(4): 253–9.

12. SM. Setta, S.D. Shemie. An explanation and analysis of how world religions formulate their ethical decisions on withdrawing treatment and determining death. *Philosophy, Ethics, and Humanities in Medicine*, 2015; 10(1): 1–22.

13. C. Sheer. Torah U-Madda and the brain death debate. In: Farber Z, editor. *Halachic realities–Collected essays on brain death*. United Kingdom: Maggid; 2015.

14. R.Y.A. Breitowitz. The brain death controversy in Jewish Law. *Jewish Law*, 2015.

15. A.C. Miller, A. Ziad-Miller, E.M. Elamin. Brain death and Islam: the interface of religion, culture, history, law, and modern medicine. *Chest*, 2014; 146(4): 1092–101.

16. R. Arbour, H.M.S. AlGhamdi, L. Peters. Islam, brain death, and transplantation: culture, faith, and jurisprudence. *AACN Advanced Critical Care*, 2012; 23(4): 381–94.

17. A. Lewis, N. Adams, A. Chopra, et al. Organ support after death by neurologic criteria in pediatric patients. *Critical Care Medicine*, 2017; 45(9): e916–24.

18. A. Lewis, N. Adams, P. Varelas, et al. Organ support after death by neurologic criteria: Results of a survey of US neurologists. *Neurology*, 2016; 87(8): 827–34.

19. A. Lewis, A. Bakkar, E. Kreiger-Benson, et al. Determination of death by neurologic criteria around the world. *Neurology*, 2020; 95(3): e299–e309.

20. L. Jacobbi, H. Franz, M.B. Coolican. HealthCare Ethics Forum '94: Organ transplantation and donation. *AACN Clinical Issues in Critical Care Nursing*, 1994; 5: 324–8.

21. H.G. Franz, W. DeJong, S.M. Wolfe, et al. Explaining brain death: A critical feature of the donation process. *Journal of Transplant Coordination*, 1997; 7(1): 14–21.

22. D.T. Savaria, M.A. Rovelli, R.T. Schweizer. Donor family surveys provide useful information for organ procurement. *Transplantation Proceedings*, 1990; 22: 316–17.

23. N. Kentish-Barnes, S. Chevret, G. Cheisson,et al. Grief symptoms in relatives who experienced organ donation requests in the ICU. *American Journal of Respiratory and Critical Care Medicine*, 2018; 198(6): 751–8.

24. S. Trevick, M. Kim, A. Naidech. Communication, leadership, and decision-making in the Neuro-ICU. *Current Neurology and Neuroscience Reports*, 2016; 16(11): 1–8.

25. P. Douglas, C. Goldschmidt, M. McCoyd, et al. Simulation-based training in brain death determination incorporating family discussion. *Journal of Graduate Medical Education*, 2018; 10(5): 553–8.

26. N. Kentish-Barnes, L.A. Siminoff, W. Walker, et al. A narrative review of family members' experience of organ donation request after brain death in the critical care setting. *Intensive Care Medicine*, 2019; 45(3): 331–42.

27. A. Lewis, P. Varelas, D. Greer. Prolonging support after brain death: When families ask for more. *Neurocritical Care*, 2016; 24(3): 481–7.

28. A.L. Flamm, M.L. Smith, P.A. Mayer. Family members' requests to extend physiologic support after declaration of brain death: A case series analysis and proposed guidelines for clinical management. *Journal of Clinical Ethics*, 2014; 25(3): 222–37.

29. J.A. Russell, L.G. Epstein, D.M. Greer, et al. Brain death, the determination of brain death, and member guidance for brain death accommodation requests. *Neurology*, 2019; 92(5): 228–32.

30. A. Lewis, P. Varelas, D.M. Greer. Controversies after brain death when families ask for more. *Chest*, 2015; 149(2): 607–8.

31. D.A. Shewmon. Chronic "brain death": Meta-analysis and conceptual consequences. *Neurology*, 1998; 51(6): 1538–45.

32. D.J. Powner, I.M. Bernstein. Extended somatic support for pregnant women after brain death. *Critical Care Medicine*, 2003; 31(4): 1241–9.

33. A. Lewis, T.M. Pope. Physician power to declare death by neurologic criteria threatened. *Neurocritical Care*, 2017; 26(3): 446–9.

34. E.J.O. Kompanje. Families and brain death. *Seminars in Neurology*, 2015; 35: 165–73.

35. A. Lewis, J. Howard, A. Watsula-Morley, et al. An educational initiative to improve medical student awareness about brain death. *Clinical Neurology and Neurosurgery*, 2018; 167: 99–105.

Index